# Models for Population Health Improvement by Health Care Systems and Partners

Tensions and Promise on the Path Upstream

PROCEEDINGS OF A WORKSHOP

Melissa Maitin-Shepard, *Rapporteur*

Roundtable on Population Health Improvement

Board on Population Health and Public Health Practice

Health and Medicine Division

*The National Academies of*
SCIENCES · ENGINEERING · MEDICINE

THE NATIONAL ACADEMIES PRESS
*Washington, DC*
**www.nap.edu**

THE NATIONAL ACADEMIES PRESS   500 Fifth Street, NW   Washington, DC 20001

This activity was supported by contracts between the National Academy of Sciences and the Association of American Medical Colleges, Blue Cross and Blue Shield of North Carolina, The California Endowment, Dartmouth-Hitchcock, Geisinger, Kaiser Permanente, The Kresge Foundation, Nemours, The Rippel Foundation/ReThink Health, Robert Wood Johnson Foundation, U.S. Department of Health and Human Services' Program Support Center, and Wake Forest Baptist Health. Any opinions, findings, conclusions, or recommendations expressed in this publication do not necessarily reflect the views of any organization or agency that provided support for the project.

International Standard Book Number-13: 978-0-309-26532-4
International Standard Book Number-10: 0-309-26532-0
Digital Object Identifier: https://doi.org/10.17226/26059

Additional copies of this publication are available from the National Academies Press, 500 Fifth Street, NW, Keck 360, Washington, DC 20001; (800) 624-6242 or (202) 334-3313; http://www.nap.edu.

Copyright 2022 by the National Academy of Sciences. All rights reserved.

Printed in the United States of America

Suggested citation: National Academies of Sciences, Engineering, and Medicine. 2022. *Models for population health improvement by health care systems and partners: Tensions and promise on the path upstream: Proceedings of a workshop.* Washington, DC: The National Academies Press. https://doi.org/10.17226/26059.

*The National Academies of*
# SCIENCES • ENGINEERING • MEDICINE

The **National Academy of Sciences** was established in 1863 by an Act of Congress, signed by President Lincoln, as a private, nongovernmental institution to advise the nation on issues related to science and technology. Members are elected by their peers for outstanding contributions to research. Dr. Marcia McNutt is president.

The **National Academy of Engineering** was established in 1964 under the charter of the National Academy of Sciences to bring the practices of engineering to advising the nation. Members are elected by their peers for extraordinary contributions to engineering. Dr. John L. Anderson is president.

The **National Academy of Medicine** (formerly the Institute of Medicine) was established in 1970 under the charter of the National Academy of Sciences to advise the nation on medical and health issues. Members are elected by their peers for distinguished contributions to medicine and health. Dr. Victor J. Dzau is president.

The three Academies work together as the **National Academies of Sciences, Engineering, and Medicine** to provide independent, objective analysis and advice to the nation and conduct other activities to solve complex problems and inform public policy decisions. The National Academies also encourage education and research, recognize outstanding contributions to knowledge, and increase public understanding in matters of science, engineering, and medicine.

Learn more about the National Academies of Sciences, Engineering, and Medicine at **www.nationalacademies.org**.

*The National Academies of*
SCIENCES • ENGINEERING • MEDICINE

**Consensus Study Reports** published by the National Academies of Sciences, Engineering, and Medicine document the evidence-based consensus on the study's statement of task by an authoring committee of experts. Reports typically include findings, conclusions, and recommendations based on information gathered by the committee and the committee's deliberations. Each report has been subjected to a rigorous and independent peer-review process and it represents the position of the National Academies on the statement of task.

**Proceedings** published by the National Academies of Sciences, Engineering, and Medicine chronicle the presentations and discussions at a workshop, symposium, or other event convened by the National Academies. The statements and opinions contained in proceedings are those of the participants and are not endorsed by other participants, the planning committee, or the National Academies.

For information about other products and activities of the National Academies, please visit www.nationalacademies.org/about/whatwedo.

## PLANNING COMMITTEE ON HEALTH CARE SYSTEM APPROACHES TO POPULATION HEALTH: TENSIONS AND PROGRESS[1]

**MARC N. GOUREVITCH** (*Chair*), Chair, Department of Population Health, New York University Langone Health
**PHILIP M. ALBERTI,** Senior Director, Health Equity Research and Policy, Association of American Medical Colleges
**SALLY A. KRAFT,** Vice President of Population Health, Dartmouth-Hitchcock Medical Center
**SANNE MAGNAN,** Senior Fellow, HealthPartners Institute
**RAHUL RAJKUMAR,** Senior Vice President and Chief Medical Officer, Blue Cross and Blue Shield of North Carolina
**LOURDES J. RODRÍGUEZ,** Senior Program Officer, St. David's Foundation

*Health and Medicine Division Staff*

**ALINA BACIU,** Roundtable Director
**CARLA ALVARADO,** Program Officer (*until January 2021*)
**BRITTANY DAVENPORT,** Senior Program Assistant (*until December 2019*)
**HARIKA DYER,** Senior Program Assistant (*from April 2020*)

---

[1] The National Academies of Sciences, Engineering, and Medicine's planning committees are solely responsible for organizing the workshop, identifying topics, and choosing speakers. The responsibility for the published Proceedings of a Workshop Series rests with the workshop rapporteur and the institution.

# ROUNDTABLE ON POPULATION HEALTH IMPROVEMENT[1]

**SANNE MAGNAN** (*Co-Chair*), Senior Fellow, HealthPartners Institute; Adjunct Assistant Professor, Division of Medicine, University of Minnesota
**JOSHUA M. SHARFSTEIN** (*Co-Chair*), Associate Dean for Public Health Practice and Training, Johns Hopkins Bloomberg School of Public Health
**PHILIP M. ALBERTI,** Senior Director, Health Equity Research and Policy, Association of American Medical Colleges
**JOHN AUERBACH,** Executive Director, Trust for America's Health
**CATHY BAASE,** Chair, Board of Directors, Michigan Health Improvement Alliance; Consultant for Health Strategy, The Dow Chemical Company
**RAYMOND BAXTER,** President and Chief Executive Officer, Blue Shield of California Foundation
**DEBBIE I. CHANG,** Senior Vice President, Policy and Prevention, Nemours
**MARC N. GOUREVITCH,** Professor and Chair, Department of Population Health, New York University Langone Health
**GARTH GRAHAM,** President, Aetna Foundation
**GARY R. GUNDERSON,** Vice President, Faith Health, School of Divinity, Wake Forest University
**WAYNE JONAS,** Executive Director, Integrative Health Programs, H&S Ventures, Samueli Foundation
**ROBERT M. KAPLAN,** Professor, Center for Advanced Study in the Behavioral Sciences, Stanford University
**DAVID A. KINDIG,** Professor Emeritus of Population Health Sciences, Emeritus Vice Chancellor for Health Sciences, School of Medicine and Public Health, University of Wisconsin–Madison
**MICHELLE LARKIN,** Associate Vice President, Associate Chief of Staff, Robert Wood Johnson Foundation
**PHYLLIS D. MEADOWS,** Senior Fellow, Health Program, The Kresge Foundation
**BOBBY MILSTEIN,** Director, ReThink Health
**JOSÉ T. MONTERO,** Director, Office for State, Tribal, Local and Territorial Support, Centers for Disease Control and Prevention
**KAREN MURPHY,** Executive Vice President and Chief Innovation

---

[1] The National Academies of Sciences, Engineering, and Medicine's forums and roundtables do not issue, review, or approve individual documents. The responsibility for the published Proceedings of a Workshop rests with the workshop rapporteur and the institution.

Officer, Founding Director, Steele Institute for Healthcare Innovation, Geisinger
**RAHUL RAJKUMAR,** Senior Vice President and Chief Medical Officer, Blue Cross and Blue Shield of North Carolina
**LOURDES J. RODRÍGUEZ,** Director, Center for Place-Based Initiatives, Dell Medical School; Associate Professor, Department of Population Health, The University of Texas at Austin
**PAMELA RUSSO,** Senior Program Officer, Robert Wood Johnson Foundation
**MYLYNN TUFTE,** State Health Officer, North Dakota Department of Health
**HANH CAO YU,** Chief Learning Officer, The California Endowment

*Health and Medicine Division Staff*

**ALINA BACIU,** Roundtable Director
**CARLA ALVARADO,** Program Officer
**BRITTANY DAVENPORT,** Senior Program Assistant (*until December 2019*)
**HARIKA DYER,** Senior Program Assistant (*from April 2020*)

*Consultant*

**MELISSA MAITIN-SHEPARD,** *Rapporteur*

# Reviewers

This Proceedings of a Workshop was reviewed in draft form by individuals chosen for their diverse perspectives and technical expertise. The purpose of this independent review is to provide candid and critical comments that will assist the National Academies of Sciences, Engineering, and Medicine in making each published proceedings as sound as possible and to ensure that it meets the institutional standards for quality, objectivity, evidence, and responsiveness to the charge. The review comments and draft manuscript remain confidential to protect the integrity of the process.

We thank the following individuals for their review of this proceedings:

**JESSIE HECOCTA,** Blue Zones Project, Healthy Klamath
**VINU ILAKKUVAN,** PoP Health, LLC

Although the reviewers listed above provided many constructive comments and suggestions, they were not asked to endorse the content of the proceedings nor did they see the final draft before its release. The review of this proceedings was overseen by **GEORGE J. ISHAM,** HealthPartners Institute. He was responsible for making certain that an independent examination of this proceedings was carried out in accordance with standards of the National Academies and that all review comments were carefully considered. Responsibility for the final content rests entirely with the rapporteur and the National Academies.

# Contents

**ACRONYMS AND ABBREVIATIONS**     xiii

**1 INTRODUCTION**     1
Workshop Objectives, 1
Organization of the Workshop and Proceedings, 3
A Metaphor for Framing the Workshop, 4

**2 OVERVIEW OF THE LANDSCAPE: TENSIONS AND
PROMISE**     5
Activities in the Health Care Sector to Improve Social Care
 and Strengthen Social Resources, 8
Opportunities for Health: Addressing Social Determinants
 of Health, 12
Audience Discussion, 16

**3 HOW LEADERSHIP AND ORGANIZATIONAL
STRUCTURE CAN ADDRESS HEALTH-RELATED
SOCIAL NEEDS AND ADVANCE HEALTH EQUITY**     19
Redesigning a Health System to Create Well Communities, 19
Enterprise-Wide Infrastructure to Advance Health Equity, 21
Audience Discussion, 22

| 4 | **DOWNSTREAM: ADDRESSING PATIENTS' HEALTH-RELATED SOCIAL NEEDS** | 25 |
|---|---|---|
| | Rush System for Health: A Case Study for Health Equity, 25 | |
| | Many Voices: One West Side, 27 | |
| | Audience Discussion, 30 | |
| 5 | **MIDSTREAM: ACCOUNTABLE HEALTH COMMUNITIES AND PARTNERSHIPS WITH HUMAN SERVICES ORGANIZATIONS** | 33 |
| | The Denver Regional Accountable Health Community, 33 | |
| | Partnerships with Area Agencies on Aging and Other Community-Based Organizations, 35 | |
| | Audience Discussion, 38 | |
| 6 | **UPSTREAM: CHANGING ENVIRONMENTS, CHANGING POLICY** | 43 |
| | Policy and Environmental Changes to Improve Health in Klamath County, Oregon, 43 | |
| | Changing the Environment to Promote Health Outside the Four Walls of the MD Anderson Cancer Center, 46 | |
| | Audience Discussion, 49 | |
| 7 | **SMALL-GROUP INTERACTIVE EXERCISE: UP/MID/DOWNSTREAM PARADIGMS IN ADVANCING POPULATION HEALTH AND HEALTH EQUITY** | 53 |
| | Instructions, 53 | |
| | Report Back, 54 | |
| 8 | **FINAL REFLECTIONS** | 57 |

**APPENDIXES**

| A | References | 61 |
|---|---|---|
| B | Workshop Agenda | 63 |
| C | Biographical Sketches of Presenters and Moderators | 67 |
| D | Small-Group Exercise: Up/Mid/Downstream Paradigms in Advancing Population Health and Health Equity | 77 |

# Acronyms and Abbreviations

| | |
|---|---|
| AAA | Area Agencies on Aging |
| AAMC | Association of American Medical Colleges |
| CBO | community-based organization |
| CIL | Center for Independent Living |
| CMMI | Center for Medicare & Medicaid Innovation |
| CMS | Centers for Medicare & Medicaid Services |
| IOM | Institute of Medicine |
| LTSS | long-term services and supports |
| n4a | National Association of Area Agencies on Aging |
| NCDHHS | North Carolina Department of Health and Human Services |
| PRAPARE | Protocol for Responding to and Assessing Patients' Assets, Risks, and Experiences |
| RFP | request for proposal |
| SDOH | social determinants of health |
| SIREN | Social Interventions Research and Evaluation Network |
| VUMC | Vanderbilt University Medical Center |

| | |
|---|---|
| WHO | World Health Organization |
| WIC | Special Supplemental Nutrition Program for Women, Infants, and Children |

# 1

# Introduction[1]

## WORKSHOP OBJECTIVES

On September 19, 2019, the Roundtable on Population Health Improvement of the National Academies of Sciences, Engineering, and Medicine hosted a public workshop in Washington, DC, titled Models for Population Health Improvement by Health Care Systems and Partners: Tensions and Promise on the Path Upstream. The term *upstream* refers to the higher levels of action to improve health. Castrucci and Auerbach (2019) classify medical services as acting downstream in improving population health, while such activities as screening and referring to social and human services are situated midstream, and the work of changing laws, policies, and regulations to improve the community conditions for health represents upstream action.

The workshop was organized by an ad hoc planning committee to discuss the growing attention to population health, from health care delivery and health insurance organizations to the social determinants of health and their individual-level manifestation as health-related social needs, such as patients' need for transportation and housing. The charge to the planning committee is provided in Box 1-1. The workshop showcased collaborative population health improvement efforts, each of which included one or more health systems. The leadership role was not always held by a health system; in some cases, it was shared with, or held by, a public health agency, human or social services agency, or community organization.

Sanne Magnan of the HealthPartners Institute stated in her opening remarks that the Roundtable on Population Health Improvement

> **BOX 1-1**
> **Workshop Statement of Task**
>
> An ad hoc planning committee will organize and convene a 1-day public workshop to discuss the growing attention from health care delivery and health insurance organizations to the social determinants of health. Trends and examples regarding health system engagement in population health ranging from individual-level patient management efforts that focus on individual-level patient social needs and "medicalize" population health[a] to more community-level interventions will be explored and discussed. The workshop will also present examples of innovative health system efforts that are focused on upstream (meso and macro) level factors, and will discuss the challenges and benefits of promoting upstream (i.e., population-level, systems, and policy-focused) approaches to population health and health equity, including the community-level infrastructure needed to support more upstream efforts. A proceedings of the presentations and discussions at the workshop will be prepared by designated rapporteurs in accordance with institutional guidelines.
>
> ---
>
> [a] Medicalization of population health generally refers to an overly clinical or medical approach to improving health or a focus on clinical solutions at the expense of or with disregard for what evidence shows are the real factors that shape health. Lantz (2019) and Woolf (2019) offer two perspectives on medicalization, and the topic is discussed in NASEM (2019a, p. 127).

provides a trusted venue for leaders in the public and private sectors to meet and discuss the tensions as well as leverage points and opportunities arising from changes in the social and political environment for achieving population health. The roundtable vision is of a

> strong, healthful, and productive society that cultivates equal opportunity and human capital, and rests on the recognition that outcomes such as improved life expectancy, quality of life, and health for all are shaped by interdependent social, economic, environmental, genetic, behavioral, and health care factors, and will require robust national and community-based actions and dependable resources to achieve it.

Magnan informed the audience that the Health and Medicine Division of the National Academies conducted two other activities related to the topic of the workshop on addressing nonmedical but health-related social needs and social determinants of health. A Proceedings of a Workshop is available from an April 2019 workshop titled Investing in Interventions That Address the Nonmedical, Health-Related Social Needs (NASEM, 2019b). A consensus study report titled *Integrating Social Care into the Delivery of Health Care: Moving Upstream to Improve the*

*Nation's Health* (NASEM, 2019a) was released in September 2019 following the workshop.[2]

The focus of this workshop, Magnan stated, would be on the evolving efforts to respond to health-related social needs in a manner that is increasingly oriented upstream (e.g., policy change) and not limited to efforts that are somewhat more downstream, namely clinic-based and individual-level interventions (e.g., behavior change). The efforts to be highlighted in the workshop also are informed by community wisdom and by learning from partners, including and especially those from outside the health system. Throughout the workshop, speakers and panelists highlighted the interwoven efforts of health systems and their many partners to move beyond what takes place in clinical settings and to collaboratively identify and respond to the needs of patients and communities.

Magnan concluded her remarks with thanks to the planning committee, which, in addition to herself, included Philip Alberti of the Association of American Medical Colleges, Marc Gourevitch of New York University Langone Health, Sally Kraft of Dartmouth-Hitchcock, Jeff Levi of The George Washington University, Rahul Rajkumar of Blue Cross and Blue Shield of North Carolina, and Lourdes Rodriguez of The University of Texas at Austin. The charge to the planning committee is provided in Box 1-1.

## ORGANIZATION OF THE WORKSHOP AND PROCEEDINGS

The workshop featured two keynote presentations (see Chapter 2) providing an overview of some of the landscape of population health improvement efforts from the perspective of health systems, including the "tensions and promise" mentioned in the workshop title. Four panel sessions and discussions followed, primarily from a health systems perspective. Programs and partnerships that were showcased focused on expanding midstream and upstream approaches to population health improvement. In Chapter 3, the first panel focused on how leadership and organizational structure can support addressing health-related social needs and advance health equity. In Chapter 4, the second panel focused on a health system and community partnership. In Chapter 5, the third panel featured a model for a health-sector partnership with a human services organization. In Chapter 6, the final panel explored changing systems and changing policy (e.g., tobacco laws). A small-group interactive exercise examining upstream, midstream, and downstream paradigms in

---

[2] That committee's report, *Integrating Social Care into the Delivery of Health Care: Moving Upstream to Improve the Nation's Health,* was released on September 25, 2019, and is available for free download at https://www.nap.edu/25467 (accessed May 28, 2021).

advancing population health and health equity is described in Chapter 7. The workshop concluded with reflections on the workshop's presentations and discussions in Chapter 8.

## A METAPHOR FOR FRAMING THE WORKSHOP

In his reflections at the close of the workshop, Bobby Milstein of ReThink Health shared a colleague's quote that "health care is a planet that thinks of itself as the sun." The speakers, Milstein asserted, illustrated a new standard for how health care institutions are working to reposition the systems that thought of themselves as the center of the universe, and that have been resourced accordingly. The workshop, he added, shares stories of how varied leaders are "marrying" health system efforts and the existing, longstanding community infrastructure of human services and other organizations.

# 2

# Overview of the Landscape: Tensions and Promise

The workshop began with two keynote presentations that provided an overview of the landscape related to how actors in the health care delivery system are addressing health-related social needs and the social determinants of health (SDOH), and it explored some of the tensions and promise of those efforts. Highlights from the two presentations and subsequent discussion are provided in Box 2-1.

Session moderator Marc Gourevitch of New York University Langone Health began by sharing a simple diagram that he used to illustrate the workshop agenda. As Figure 2-1 shows, different categories of organizations may be better suited to assume a lead or a partner role when working to respond to the spectrum of social needs, depending on whether those needs are expressed by patients or by communities. Gourevitch pointed out that the gradient from downstream to upstream interventions is a continuum, and any single action such as screening or referral could be viewed as downstream or midstream depending on whether one is approaching it from the perspective of a health system or a community-based organization. The boundaries among categories are fluid as well, and as one moves up or down in the figure, the role of any particular sector shifts. For example, Gourevitch noted that health care would be more likely to be in the lead on a downstream (e.g., clinically oriented) effort, and to assume a more supportive, collaborative role in an upstream effort, which may be better led by a social service agency.

Gourevitch explained that one of the workshop's tasks was to showcase examples of interventions from across the spectrum that feature dif-

> **BOX 2-1**
> **Key Points Made by Individual Speakers and Participants**
>
> - Some organizations are best suited to lead and others to partner or collaborate in addressing downstream, midstream, and upstream factors regarding health-related social needs or social determinants of health (SDOH). (Gourevitch)
> - There is a lack of consensus regarding which social risk factors are most important to screen for in clinical settings, which measures to use in screening for those factors, and even whether conducting social risk screenings at the patient level is appropriate. (Gottlieb)
> - There are five categories (five As) of SDOH-related health-sector activities—awareness (which can be individually and/or community focused), adjustment and assistance (which are individually focused), and alignment and advocacy (which are community focused). (Gottlieb, in reference to NASEM, 2019a)
> - As part of focusing on greater integration of social services in health care, it is important to keep in mind potential unintended consequences (e.g., on patients, clinicians, the social sector), but early research indicates some of the feared negative consequences may be unlikely. (Gottlieb)
> - Safety net providers frequently adjust medical care to accommodate social factors that could interfere with treatment, although this is not systematically built into all health care practices. (Gottlieb)
> - North Carolina's Healthy Opportunities initiative pilots will allow the state to examine how contributions to social services may improve health care outcomes. (Money)
> - It is important to listen to communities and align activities with community needs and priorities. An initiative is more likely to be successful when the community is invested in the solution and the outcome. (Money)

|  | HEALTH CARE/HEALTH SYSTEM | PUBLIC HEALTH AGENCY | HUMAN/SOCIAL SERVICES/OTHER SECTOR ORG |
|---|---|---|---|
| Downstream | Lead | Partner | Partner |
| Midstream | Partner | Lead or Partner | Lead or Partner |
| Upstream | Partner | Lead or Partner | Lead or Partner |

**FIGURE 2-1** Heuristic illustrating the roles of various sectors in downstream, midstream, and upstream interventions.
SOURCE: Gourevitch presentation, September 19, 2019.

ferent types of entities, including a public health agency, health system, and human services agency in the lead role. Much of the discussion would feature the perspectives of health systems or health care organizations. The examples are intended to illustrate the range of innovative work taking place across the country and elevate the types of governance, leadership, and institutional infrastructure that are needed to help health systems work with communities and other partners to address health and the nonhealth needs of their patients and communities.

Gourevitch also described Figure 2-2 as a map of some of the lead conceptual models that situate health care's contribution to population health on the downstream, midstream, and upstream continuum. He noted that the diagram references recent key publications from Alderwick and Gottlieb (2019), Auerbach (2016), Castrucci and Auerbach (2019), and Kindig and Isham (2014), and it aims to portray commonalities and highlight differences in language and framing across types of interventions. As he explained, moving from the bottom to the top, attention shifts from downstream to midstream to upstream. From left to right are

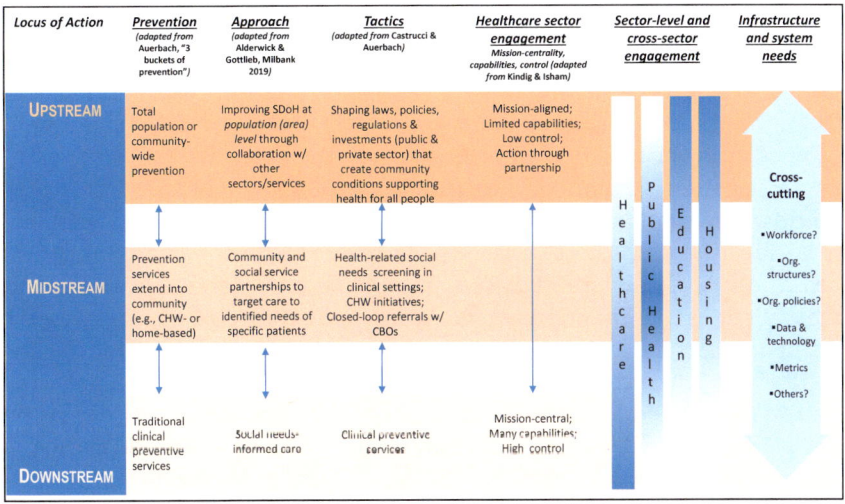

**FIGURE 2-2** Diagram displaying up/mid/downstream paradigms in advancing population health and health equity.
NOTES: The bidirectional arrows illustrate the recognition that practices or activities do not fall neatly in one category but occur on a spectrum. The gradations of color among the few sectors provided as illustration (health care, public health, education, and housing) are meant to signify the level of responsibility for a given sector (darker = greater; lighter = lesser).
SOURCE: Gourevitch presentation, September 19, 2019. Prepared with assistance from Alina Baciu.

various models or frameworks that address contributions of health care, public health, and other sectors (see narrow blue bands at right) along the spectrum from identifying and addressing an individual's risk factors to tackling upstream SDOH.

## ACTIVITIES IN THE HEALTH CARE SECTOR TO IMPROVE SOCIAL CARE AND STRENGTHEN SOCIAL RESOURCES

Via videoconference, Laura Gottlieb of the Social Interventions Research and Evaluation Network (SIREN), University of California, San Francisco, presented on ways health care systems are identifying and intervening in social conditions as part of efforts to improve health for individual patients and communities. She suggested that the recent emphasis on addressing SDOH and social risks within the health care delivery system is only one part of a comprehensive strategy necessary to achieve population health and health equity.

### Categories of Health Care Activities Related to Social Conditions

Gottlieb explained that the National Academies of Sciences, Engineering, and Medicine's Committee on Integrating Social Needs Care into the Delivery of Health Care to Improve the Nation's Health, of which she was a member, articulated five categories of health-sector activities related to providing social care or improving social conditions—the five As (awareness, adjustment, assistance, alignment, and advocacy; NASEM, 2019a). A foundational step for improving social conditions is increasing awareness of social risk and protective factors. As a result, an increasing number of health care systems are investing in ways to obtain that information at the patient and population levels. At the patient level, examples include standardized social risk screening tools such as measures proposed by the National Academies committee;[1] the National Association of Community Health Centers and partners' Protocol for Responding to and Assessing Patients' Assets, Risks, and Experiences (PRAPARE) tool;[2] and the social risk domains included in a tool developed under the Center for Medicare & Medicaid Innovation's (CMMI's) Accountable Health Communities demonstration project. She noted that there is a lack of consensus regarding which social risk factors are most important to screen for in

---

[1] The committee authored the report *Integrating Social Needs Care into the Delivery of Health Care*, available at https://www.nap.edu/25467 (accessed July 1, 2020).
[2] The National Association of Community Health Centers' PRAPARE assessment tool is available at http://www.nachc.org/research-and-data/prapare/about-the-prapare-assessment-tool (accessed July 1, 2020).

clinical settings, which measures to use in screening for those factors, and even whether conducting social risk screenings at the patient level is appropriate.

One alternative to collecting patient information involves using community-level social risk data as a proxy for individual level risks, such as by linking a patient's address or zip code with census tract data. As Gottlieb explained, several new technologies can be useful in displaying community-level data. For example, HealthLandscape allows health systems to map data on where their patients live and the social resources that are available in that area.

Just as awareness strategies span the spectrum from a focus on the individual patient to a focus on the whole community, Gottlieb explained that health care system activities to intervene in social conditions are also wide ranging. Two categories of activities that focus on patients and the delivery of health care services are (1) the adjustment of medical care or treatment decisions based on information about social risk, and (2) interventions by health care systems to assist patients in improving social conditions by providing social services onsite or connecting patients to social services offsite. Gottlieb explained that many providers working in safety net health care delivery systems already adjust medical care to accommodate individual-level social factors that could interfere with treatment, although these alterations are not always done systematically. Adjustments can be made to improve access, diagnostics, or treatment. For example, to improve access to care, health care systems use mobile units, offer clinics on evenings and weekends, provide interpreter services, and adjust written resources for different literacy levels.

The American College of Obstetricians and Gynecologists guideline on preeclampsia includes "low-income" as a moderate risk factor and suggests it be used to guide aspirin therapy. As another example, providers may opt to avoid using diuretics when treating hypertension in people without housing given challenges with restroom access. Gottlieb also described innovative work on diabetes care informed by social risk. For example, a 2019 paper explored ways in which providers change the way they care for patients with diabetes based on information about the patient's social risk (Hessler et al., 2019). She noted the study found that providers reported changing blood sugar goals, engaging in more cost-sensitive prescribing, and making other treatment changes based on information about social risk. She suggested that this model could also help to inform chronic disease management in other areas.

She pointed out that the health care system has not yet determined what interventions work best for which populations, and care informed by social risk is applied inconsistently. She specified that a major challenge to adjustment strategies is that the health care system has not clarified how to implement some of these recommendations nor elucidated what interventions work best for which populations. Gottlieb suggested that more research is needed to enable the use of social risk data to improve medical care, social risk data should be available to providers at the point of care, and effective interventions should be built into electronic health systems.

Gottlieb went on to describe "social risk-targeted care," which involves using health care system resources to improve patients' social context. In the National Academies report, these activities are categorized as "assistance" strategies. Examples include helping patients obtain a refrigerator to be able to refrigerate medications, connecting patients to food programs, and helping patients obtain jobs paying a living wage.

In addition to the patient-directed adjustment and assistance strategies, Gottlieb noted that the National Academies committee also considered ways that the health care system can affect social conditions at the community level. Strategies include better aligning health care actions with community priorities and advocating for policy changes that change the resource and equity landscape. Examples include ways hospitals and health care systems align their own institutional practices around issues, such as procurement and hiring, with the needs of the surrounding community. Another example is CMMI's Accountable Health Communities demonstration project, in which 24 health systems are supported to convene intersectoral advisory committees to fill gaps in social service needs.

Gottlieb used the issue of food security to illustrate how the five As could complement one another—and potentially be deployed simultaneously. For example, screening for food insecurity in health care settings is increasingly common. Providers could use that information to adjust insulin doses for patients with food insecurity when food access is low. Community health workers could assist by providing support for meal programs or connect patients with existing programs. Hospitals could align their needs with those of the community by sourcing hospital food from local farms or hosting farmers' markets. They could also advocate for increased or sustained food program benefits for low-income populations. Figure 2-3 outlines these five categories of SDOH-related health-sector activities.

### Tensions on the Path Upstream

Gottlieb stated that while both downstream and upstream approaches to increasing health care system engagement are critical, there are many obstacles to achieving them; just as importantly, there is the potential that such approaches may incur unintended consequences. One potential unintended consequence that Gottlieb highlighted is that

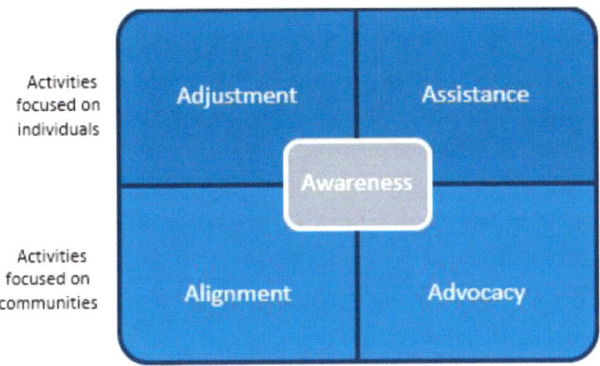

**FIGURE 2-3** The five As: A visual representation of the categories of SDOH-related health-sector activities.
SOURCES: Gottlieb presentation, September 19, 2019; NASEM (2019a, Figure 2-1, p. 34).

asking about social risk factors could offend patients, worsening relationships with the health care system and exacerbating inequities in access to health care services or treatment adherence. She highlighted new work suggesting that this may be an unlikely effect, but she noted that this area requires more study. Another potential unintended consequence is the possibility that if not monitored, the availability of social risk data at the point of care could increase medical treatment bias and discrimination. Gottlieb also wondered "could the health care sector's sudden enthusiasm around SDOH actually end up exacerbating our underfunding crisis in the third sector?"[3] She suggested that academics, patients, providers, community members, public health practitioners, and social services representatives work together to increase awareness of potential unintended consequences and invest in effectiveness and implementation research to understand how health care sector activities affect patients from different demographic groups, as well as caregivers, and the social sector.

Gottlieb noted that initial research from SIREN has produced early evidence that some of the potential unintended consequences described are unlikely. For example, her research group has found that many, although not all, patients appreciate being asked about social risk in clinical settings. It also found that patients want to talk about social risks in health care settings, even if they do not expect health care providers to

---

[3] The *third sector*, or *social sector*, is an umbrella term for organizations that are neither in the public nor private sectors, such as community volunteer organizations and other nonprofit organizations.

resolve the issues. Also, health care providers in clinics that provide more social services are less likely to be burned out.

Gottlieb noted that research from SIREN could help to inform organizations working to improve the way health care systems engage around social conditions as a strategy for improving health.

## OPPORTUNITIES FOR HEALTH: ADDRESSING SOCIAL DETERMINANTS OF HEALTH

E. Benjamin Money of the North Carolina Department of Health and Human Services (NCDHHS) spoke about the state's approach to addressing SDOH. He opened by noting that he is relatively new to his current role and previously led the primary care association in North Carolina, which was an early partner in addressing social determinants, or social drivers, of health. Money noted that most of the current work builds on successful past initiatives.

### Background on North Carolina and Its Approach to Addressing Social Drivers of Health

Money provided background on the state of North Carolina, noting that it is the 10th most populous state in the United States and 37th in overall health status. Approximately one in five children experience food insecurity and a similar number have two or more adverse childhood events. Nearly half (47 percent) of women experience intimate partner violence. The state's legislature has not expanded Medicaid, which would benefit more than 500,000 people. He noted that 29 percent of low-income adults have forgone needed care because of cost. Money pointed out that North Carolina also has challenges with affordable housing and growing gentrification in urban areas, which are particularly affecting people displaced from coastal areas due to hurricanes. Politically, North Carolina is "purple," with a Democratic governor and a Republican-led legislature. The state is also racially diverse.

As Money pointed out, the state of North Carolina has recognized the importance of purchasing *health*, rather than just *health care*, as health is driven by more than health care. In fact, Money stated, health care accounts for only 10 percent of health status, and health is instead largely determined by behaviors, social circumstances, and environmental exposures. As most of the state's health-related spending is on health care, there is a significant opportunity to increase attention to the other factors that influence health.

The state's vision for addressing social drivers of health involves optimizing health and well-being for all residents by bridging communities and the health care system. Money pointed out that achieving this vision will require partnerships and humility. The state is focused on partnering with community-engaged organizations and moving into managed care. As he explained, North Carolina is the largest state without a Medicaid managed care program. The state is moving from a fee-for-service model to one that is value based and takes a whole-person approach to care, integrates physical and behavioral health care, and seeks to buy health rather than health care. He noted that the state is taking a data-centered approach to this work.

## Medicaid Transformation

Money explained that Medicaid transformation is a key driver of the state's work to address social factors that influence health. He noted that Medicaid transformation was originally scheduled to launch in February 2020, but political disagreements around Medicaid expansion between the governor and legislature are likely to delay that timeline.[4] The state is intending to move toward a "whole-person care system" with Medicaid managed care organizations, also called prepaid health plans. These prepaid health plans will focus on physical health, behavioral health, and unmet social needs using a three-tiered provider structure. The system will move toward increased value by providing enhanced payments and supports for the provider to engage in case management and care coordination. Money outlined three components of the Healthy Opportunities landscape: (1) implementing Healthy Opportunity pilots that are part of the state's 1115 waiver from the Centers for Medicare & Medicaid Services, (2) incorporating robust elements within Medicaid managed care, and (3) using a Healthy Opportunities framework for all populations. Priority domains for case management and value-based payments include food security, housing stability, transportation, interpersonal environment, employment, toxic stress, and adverse childhood experiences. Money outlined the elements of the Medicaid managed care model, as shown in Figure 2-4.

The Healthy Opportunities initiative pilots will allow the state to examine how contributions to discrete services may improve health care outcomes. In-depth analysis of the strategies and results will drive future adjustments to the Medicaid managed care model. A key component of the

---

[4] The transition to Mediaid Managed Care is expected to take place in summer 2021. See https://files.nc.gov/ncdma/NCMT_Provider_FactSheet-NCMT-Overview_20210118.pdf (accessed May 4, 2021) and https://journalnow.com/governor-signs-medicaid-transformation-bill-new-format-projected-to-start-in-july-2021/article_7379d2f5-8830-5ffc-8f67-7889d7fef742.html for more information (accessed May 4, 2021).

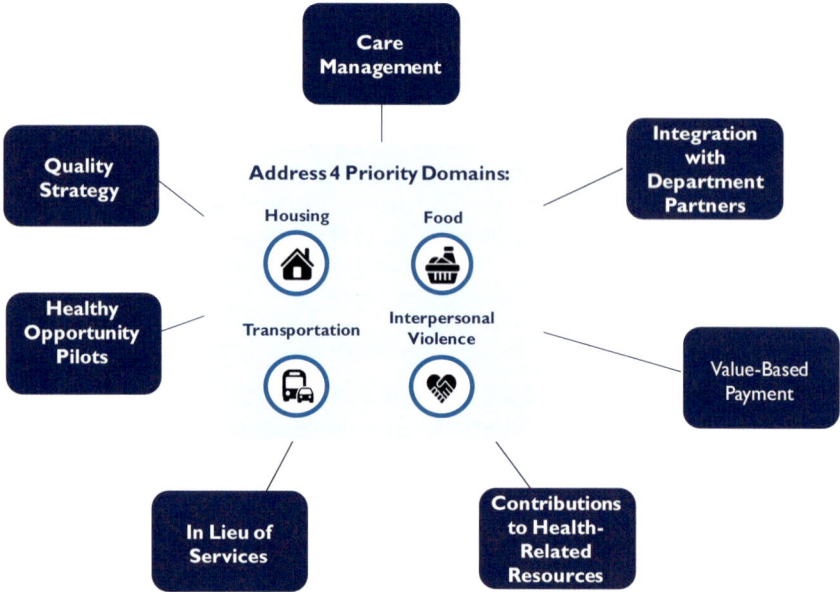

**FIGURE 2-4** Visual representation of the elements, including four priority domains, in North Carolina's Medicaid managed care program.
SOURCE: Money presentation, September 19, 2019.

model will be care management that uses teams of care managers focused on navigating and providing resources for social services and trauma-informed care. As Money explained, the model will use an interdisciplinary team-based care approach that includes providers such as housing and legal specialists. Standardized screening tools and an electronic referral system will also be used. Greater attention will be given to high-needs cases, such as people experiencing homelessness or interpersonal violence.

The program is also focused on aligning payments and incentives. Money pointed out that value-based payments for health and the delivery of social services create incentives for prepaid health plans to invest in those services, particularly in communities involved in the pilots. Infrastructure and elements of the program include

- geo-mapping hotspots of social drivers across the state,
- standardized statewide screening questions on SDOH that were adapted from existing tools such as PRAPARE and tested within the state,
- a statewide coordinated care network with a shared technology platform called NCCARE360, and

- community health workers that are trained through community colleges statewide to be employed by health systems and health plans.

As of May 2021, the NCCARES360 website indicated that 100 counties in the state had joined the coordinated care network.[5] In addition, Money noted that a statewide resource directory is being developed. While a statewide call center has existed for several years, the resource directory will be integrated into the call center and data will be collected and analyzed. The Unite Us referral platform will also be made available and supported by county-level community engagement managers. In the future, Money explained, the state intends to be able to use data obtained through the resource platform on social needs and morbidity data through the health information exchange for data analytics and geo-mapping.

## Healthy Opportunities Pilot Program

Money described the Healthy Opportunities pilot program, which will dedicate $650 million over 5 years to pay for discrete services to enhance health outcomes for Medicaid beneficiaries in managed care plans. The prepaid health plans would provide this funding through lead pilot entities, which are organizations that bridge the relationship between health care organizations and housing, food, and transportation service providers in the community. Money noted that it will be important to ensure that the pilot pays for nonhealth care interventions that will improve the health of the most vulnerable patients, and that the services are used. To be eligible for the program, participants must have at least one physical or behavioral health condition and one social risk factor. Examples of eligible physical or behavioral health conditions include pregnant women with a multiple pregnancy (i.e., twins or more), children in neonatal intensive care units, and adults with two or more chronic conditions. Social risk factors include homelessness, food insecurity, and transportation insecurity. Program services must address food, housing, transportation, or interpersonal violence. For example, services to address housing could include assistance with 1 month's rent, security deposit, utilities, or weatherization programs. Services to address food insecurity could include support with enrollment in the Special Supplemental Nutrition Program for Women, Infants, and Children or the Supplemental Nutrition Assistance Program, healthy food packages, and medically tailored meals for people with chronic disease. Transportation assistance could provide services for health care and social service visits.

---

[5] See https://nccare360.org (accessed May 27, 2021).

With respect to financing, Money explained, prepaid health plans will have a capitated rate and advanced care payments with incentives that move toward value and incorporate social drivers that influence health. To evaluate the effect, the state has partnered with the University of North Carolina and the Sheps Center for Health Services Research. The evaluation will involve rapid cycle assessments that quickly determine which strategies are working and allow for adjustments as needed. The goal is to ensure that the program works with communities and meets their needs. Models will be used to expand the approach statewide.

The development of the program is under way, with review of the request for proposals (RFP) and final revisions to program details taking place during fall 2019. After the RFP is released, funding for lead pilot entities was intended to be awarded in early 2020.[6] For the next 5 years, the focus will be on building the capacity of the lead pilot entities, health services organizations, and communities, as well as refining the model. The program is slated to end in October 2024.

In addition to NCDHHS, other key partners include the state's Medicaid program, Blue Cross and Blue Shield of North Carolina, several health systems within the state, and primary care providers that have already been participating in the Medicare Shared Savings Program and other value-based payment models.

## AUDIENCE DISCUSSION

Gourevitch opened the audience discussion by asking Gottlieb if her research has found effective approaches based on the five As of care informed by social risk. Gottlieb responded that research has been primarily focused on awareness and assistance activities. Research on adjustment strategies exists in select medical disciplines but has not been collected and aggregated specifically under this bucket. Though there is considerable interest and investment in alignment and advocacy strategies, there has not been much research done in these areas. This is in part because it is more difficult to conduct research in a multisectoral partnership, which is more common with those types of interventions. Gottlieb suggested that more health services research on all of these topics is needed.

Gourevitch asked Money to what extent the health care sector is in support of, and engaged with, the programs in North Carolina that he described. Money responded that the health care sector has been engaged

---

[6] The evaluation of proposals was suspended in May 2020 due to the COVID-19 pandemic and in January 2021 NCDHHS stated that awards would be announced in March 2021. See https://www.ncdhhs.gov/about/department-initiatives/healthy-opportunities/healthy-opportunities-pilots (accessed May 27, 2021).

from the beginning. The Medicaid transformation initiative stems from an interest by the legislature during a prior administration to move Medicaid from fee-for-service to managed care. He explained that the health care systems at that time indicated an interest in addressing factors outside their usual focus that improve health, as such factors influence health plans' abilities to improve health outcomes, which is central to a capitated payment model. When the current governor began his administration, the model shifted to emphasize SDOH and the Healthy Opportunities pilot was developed. Health systems, providers, and other community members were invited to comment on the model for the Healthy Opportunities pilot, which was subsequently adjusted based on public feedback.

Sanne Magnan of the HealthPartners Institute asked how to ensure that systems in communities address community needs rather than assess risk. Money responded by emphasizing the importance of listening to communities and aligning activities with community needs and priorities. He noted that public health often uses its own data sets, analytics, and geomaps to identify the problems and the solutions, ignoring the community's own perceived needs and proposed solutions. He pointed out that an initiative is more likely to be successful when the community is invested in the solution and the outcome. Money suggested that greater emphasis on ensuring that interventions meet the needs of the community and the public health agenda fits into the community's agenda. He also pointed to the need for increased respect for the work that communities have done and leadership within the community.

Gottlieb added that she agreed with Money that it is important to ensure that health care delivery interventions meet the needs of patients and communities. For example, she noted that some research has shown that people who agree with the idea of social risk factors do not consistently accept assistance from health care systems related to these risk factors. Gottlieb noted that this reveals an important research question about how health care systems can ensure that any new activity meets patients' needs and priorities.

Jennifer Little of Klamath County Public Health in Oregon asked Money how the programs and frameworks that he described, such as the Healthy Opportunities pilots, may work differently in rural versus urban environments. Money responded by noting that North Carolina is both an urban and a rural state, and these types of communities have different needs. For example, a rural transportation system is different from an urban one. He noted that the state's Office of Rural Health works with rural counties on approaches to address the four domains (see Figure 2-4) at the county level. For example, Money described a community health center in the more rural eastern part of the state that has used existing resources, such as church and agency vans, to create a transportation network. They also developed community gardens to address food insecurity. A faith-based organization is supporting income development and sustainable agriculture by training community residents to become beekeepers. Money added that the closure of many critical access hospitals in rural areas provides an opportunity to determine what rural health care should look like, incorporating strategies that address the social drivers of health. Gottlieb noted that assistance is the one of the five As that would most likely differ between urban and rural populations, since urbanicity often affects resource availability.

Lourdes Rodriguez of the Dell Medical School at The University of Texas at Austin asked for the panelists' perspectives on moving from a pilot project to a scaled-up intervention. Money responded that data will be critical for demonstrating that investment in an intervention is cost saving. For example, he explained that the cost of a refrigerator for insulin is less than the cost of even an ambulance ride to the hospital for a person with diabetes who does not take his or her insulin. Gottlieb added that there could be many additional considerations, given that standard insulin does not need refrigeration if used within 28 days. An alternative cost-effective adjustment strategy for providers might be to prescribe a supply of insulin that does not require refrigeration, though the comparative effectiveness (e.g., on quality of life, adherence, and other health-related outcomes) and cost-effectiveness of these different types of interventions should be evaluated. She noted that the National Academies report on integrating social care into health care delivery includes content regarding financing strategies and how to scale up pilot projects (NASEM, 2019a).

Alyssa Crawford of Mathematica stated that interventions in health care often target the easier problems first and she sees a similar pattern emerging with interventions to address SDOH. She said longer-term investments are needed that address more challenging issues such as systemic racism and social isolation. Crawford asked the presenters about promising practices that address these types of larger challenges. Money noted that some European countries may provide a model for the United States in promoting equity in health outcomes. He stated that income inequality is a particular challenge in the United States and a lot of it stems from historic and systemic racism.

# 3

# How Leadership and Organizational Structure Can Address Health-Related Social Needs and Advance Health Equity

The first panel, moderated by Philip Alberti of the Association of American Medical Colleges (AAMC), featured two speakers who spoke about how leadership and structure can support the work of addressing social and community needs beyond clinical care. The panel was intended to address how health care organizations can coordinate and organize these types of activities in a cohesive, effective, iterative, and evaluated manner. As Alberti explained, a goal could be coordinating and integrating siloed groups in an organization focused on community-partnered science, conducting community health needs assessments, and population health management, for example. A health care organization, he added, should "have its own internal house in order" in order to be an effective partner in a multisectoral collaboration to address health and health care inequities.

Highlights from the two presentations and subsequent discussion are provided in Box 3-1.

## REDESIGNING A HEALTH SYSTEM TO CREATE WELL COMMUNITIES

Benjamin Carter of Trinity Health described what his organization is doing to manage and balance the ongoing tension between being a provider-based system with episodic health care management, population health management, and community health and well-being.

As Carter explained, Trinity Health is a $19.3 billion Catholic health care organization based in Livonia, Michigan. The organization operates

> **BOX 3-1**
> **Key Points Made by Individual Speakers and Participants**
>
> - A health care organization must "have its own internal house in order" in order to be an effective partner in a multisectoral collaborative to address health and health care inequities. (Alberti)
> - There is a need to better include and reflect the voices of the community in the design of programs and activities. Health systems' work with communities often involves a "helicopter" approach (i.e., sporadic, short-lived) rather than true investment in communities (e.g., in hiring, engagement in decision making). (Wilkins)
> - Making health equity part of the organization's mission, a priority of the board of directors (with firm commitments and accountability), and integrated into incentive systems led to increased investment in, and effect on, community health. (Carter)
> - With a large, siloed organization, leadership support and commitment (with a health equity metric as part of executive-level incentives and performance goals) and organizational structure (with institutional investment in an Office of Health Equity and related education and training) are precursors to influencing culture. (Wilkins)
> - Health care systems can engage in advocacy at the federal and state levels, as well as in shareholder advocacy to influence companies in their investment portfolio to align with their priorities. (Carter)

in 19 regions across 22 states. Its mission, which was established in 2013 when Catholic Health East and Trinity came together to form Trinity Health, is to be transformative and healing in the communities it serves. Its vision is to be a people-centered health system that delivers on the triple aim of better health, better care, and lower cost for individuals, populations, and communities. Its three core services are (1) episodic care, meaning fee-for-service care provided to individuals; (2) population health, which involves creating incentives to move to value-based care and alternative payment models; and (3) community health and well-being.

Trinity Health's journey toward a well community has three focus areas: (1) transform communities through policy, systems, and environmental changes; (2) ensure care delivery models that assess and address the needs of vulnerable patients; and (3) expand use and availability of community-based services. As Carter explained, the organization also has three main strategic initiatives. The first is to address the social influences on health, which involves tackling at least one social influence of health in each community. The other two strategic initiatives are to reduce tobacco use and obesity across the health care system.

Carter described how Trinity Health is investing in policy, systems, and environmental change strategies to improve health. Its Transforming Communities Initiative began in March 2016 and operates in eight locations, providing $18 million in grants, which has resulted in $7 million in matching funds at the community level and $40 million in community loan investments. The program addresses social influencers such as housing, food, and transportation. Trinity Health operates the initiatives in collaboration with several national technical assistance partners.

For example, as Carter explained, to address food deserts and lack of food access in Springfield, Massachusetts, where 100 percent of students qualify for free or reduced-price meals, Trinity partnered with Sodexo and the Springfield public schools to create a $21 million culinary and nutrition center. Another example of a community partnership is the Wellspring Greenhouse, which provides local fresh produce for hospital operations.

Carter concluded by outlining Trinity Health's four areas of focus in addressing health equity: (1) assess the delivery of equitable care; (2) develop equity plans; (3) provide cultural competency education; and (4) reflect the diversity of our communities, which the organization strives to do through employment, vendor relationships, and purchasing.

## ENTERPRISE-WIDE INFRASTRUCTURE TO ADVANCE HEALTH EQUITY

Consuelo H. Wilkins of the Meharry-Vanderbilt Alliance, the Vanderbilt University Medical Center (VUMC), and the Meharry Medical College, spoke about VUMC's approach to health equity. The health system began by exploring what it was already doing related to community health and health equity as part of a project with AAMC. As Wilkins explained, the research identified more than 180 internal programs and initiatives involving research, education, and community engagement focused on community health and health equity. When leaders in population health, diversity and inclusion, academic medicine, and nursing from across the health system gathered to discuss the existing health equity initiatives, they recognized that many of them were siloed and disconnected. Wilkins noted that one result of the discussions was the realization that the voices of the community needed to be included and reflected in the design of the system's programs and activities. She lamented that much of VUMC's work with communities could be viewed as a "helicopter" approach (i.e., short-lived or sporadic) rather than true, sustained investment in communities (e.g., in hiring practices and in engaging the community in decision making).

Wilkins described how VUMC has taken an enterprise-wide approach to addressing health disparities and advancing health equity. Earlier in

2019, the health system launched a new office of health equity intended to bring together education, training, research, community, and population health efforts from across the enterprise. Wilkins noted that this institutional investment in health equity is critical to the initiative's success.

With respect to education and training of health professionals, VUMC is working to ensure that all health professionals across specialties have expertise in health equity. With respect to research, the health system is working to better understand social risks and the social determinants of health and how they can be addressed, as well as the intersection between genetics and race as a social construct.

Within VUMC, the enterprise is considering how best to support the diverse 24,000 VUMC employees who have varying needs, priorities, social risks, and incomes. As an example of strong institutional commitment, Wilkins described how a health equity metric would be part of the executives' performance goals and incentive plans across mission areas.

## AUDIENCE DISCUSSION

Alberti began the audience discussion by pointing out that in the case of Trinity Health, the mission drove the infrastructure, strategy, and planning, while with VUMC, the organization's new structure created a culture of health equity across the institution. He asked Carter and Wilkins the "chicken and egg" question of whether culture or structure should come first. Carter responded that in the case of Trinity Health, as a faith-based and provider-driven organization, community health and health equity have always been part of the mission. From a financial perspective, the organization invests in community benefit ministry, which includes the unfunded costs of Medicaid. However, he pointed out that community health was not receiving the attention and focus needed to make an improvement in the communities being served. In 2013, Trinity Health adopted a mission to be transformative, which drove it to approach community health, well-being, and health equity in a different way, which would involve firm commitments, accountability, and ongoing consideration of the effect on the community. Carter noted that having health equity as part of the organization's mission and a priority of the board of directors and incentive systems was what made a difference regarding investment in—and the improvement of—community health.

Wilkins stated that, for her organization, structure was the vehicle for changing the culture. She suggested that with a relatively large, siloed organization like VUMC, it would be difficult to influence the culture without both leadership support and organizational structure. Wilkins noted that changing the culture internally has been more challenging than forming relationships with the community.

Wilkins described several barriers to institutional change. For example, academic leaders were pleased with the curriculum, yet there was student demand to add a health equity certificate program. As another example, VUMC provided grant funding for community organizations, but required them to complete detailed forms and pay up front for expenses. Wilkins suggested that changes to the culture are needed to remove barriers such as these. She pointed out that a wellness program designed for people who, for example, can afford child care and have not struggled with food insecurity may not work for people facing these and other social factors. She concluded by emphasizing that the structure provides the opportunity to change the culture through access to, and incentives for, leadership support.

Alberti asked Carter and Wilkins which person or entity at each of their organizations is accountable for the outcomes of their health equity work and how each of the stakeholders are involved in the development of metrics and incentives that are meaningful for all. Wilkins responded that at VUMC, her position is partially responsible for the outcomes of the work, and executive-level incentives and performance goals provide additional accountability. She would like for the community to do more to hold VUMC accountable for investing in projects that meet the community's needs, including them in decision-making processes, and hiring from the community.

Carter noted that at Trinity Health, the board holds the organization accountable by requiring that 25 percent of the organization's strategic plan be related to community health and well-being, equal to the weight given to financial success. The executives of all 19 regions have the same goals related to community health and well-being as the chief executive officer. In addition, there is a senior vice president for community health who is on the executive leadership team and vice presidents in each region responsible for objectives related to community health and well-being locally. Carter pointed out that much of the community health work is accomplished through partnerships.

Building on Alberti's question about accountability, Sally Kraft of Dartmouth-Hitchcock asked about what accountability measures are being used and whether there are community health metrics. She noted that many factors outside of the health system may influence a community's health status. Wilkins responded that, as a first step, VUMC is focused on identifying which measures are being used, or could be used, to collect data, using its employees as the sample population. The health system is working to develop metrics in all mission areas, including students' competencies, knowledge, and willingness to work in underserved areas, and exploring better ways to integrate into students' work the perspectives of the communities served.

Carter noted that Trinity Health has objective measurable outcomes related to issues such as reducing tobacco use and obesity. The health system uses electronic medical records to determine the extent to which it is making a difference in these areas. There is also a new metric related to social influences on health. Trinity Health uses process measures to assess its effect in the community in areas where it works in collaboration with community partners.

John Auerbach of Trust for America's Health asked Carter and Wilkins whether their organizations have considered advocating for policy change at the federal, state, and local levels. Auerbach pointed out that in his experience as a former state health official, health systems were effective advocates, but often they did not prioritize policies that would improve overall health in the state. Carter responded that Trinity Health has been active in advocacy at the federal and state levels, including calling for legislation to increase the minimum tobacco sales age to 21, change opioid prescribing, increase housing access, and address gun violence. Given its large investment portfolio, the organization also engages in shareholder advocacy to influence companies such as CVS and Walmart to align with its priorities.

Mylynn Tufte of the North Dakota Department of Health asked Carter and Wilkins about how the language used can influence the level of support among people in their organizations who are not well versed in issues related to health equity. Wilkins responded that she sometimes uses different language to communicate about her work with different audiences within the medical center. She also pointed out that different communities may face different issues and use different words to describe their resources and needs.

# 4

# Downstream: Addressing Patients' Health-Related Social Needs

Session moderator Sally Kraft of Dartmouth-Hitchcock opened the second panel session by explaining that it would showcase an outstanding partnership between Rush University Medical Center (Rush) and a coalition of organizations on the West Side of Chicago. The presentations would address the keys to successful partnership between a health system and community organizations. Highlights from the two presentations and subsequent discussion are provided in Box 4-1.

## RUSH SYSTEM FOR HEALTH: A CASE STUDY FOR HEALTH EQUITY

Darlene Oliver Hightower from Rush began her presentation with some background on the health system. As she explained, Rush is a 180-year-old medical center located on the West Side of Chicago. With 10,000 employees and $2 billion in resources, it is the largest private employer on the West Side. In 2016, Rush changed its mission to focus on improving the health of the individuals in the diverse communities it serves. As Hightower pointed out, this involved improving the quality of care for its patients and community programs, partnerships, and interventions. The strategy to execute the mission included developing deeper community partnerships.

Rush also completed its community health needs assessment in 2016, which revealed significant gaps in life expectancy among neighborhoods in Chicago. As Figure 4-1 shows, Hightower pointed out that life expectancy ranged from age 85 in downtown Chicago to age 69 in West Garfield

> **BOX 4-1**
> **Key Points Made by Individual Speakers and Participants**
>
> - In serving as an anchor institution, Rush University Medical Center (Rush) intentionally and strategically invested in the West Side of Chicago by considering its hiring practices, career paths, construction projects, supply chain, partnerships, vendors, investment in community economic development, and engagement of employees to volunteer in the surrounding community. In addition to using its own resources, by forming a collaborative, Rush could engage and persuade other health care institutions to make similar investments. (Hightower)
> - It was important both for Rush and for the community members that they be involved in the decision-making processes. (Jaco)
> - Trust between health systems and communities is important for realizing lasting change. (Kraft)
> - The lived experience that community members bring should be recognized and valued. (Jaco)
> - Factors key to the success of the health system–community partnership have included health institutions' intentionality and honesty about the role they have played in perpetuating and then addressing the disparities, having a well-known and well-respected health system champion, leveraging the power of the community, and bringing in resources from different sectors. (Jaco)
> - It is important to provide orientation and set expectations for health system executives around why community members want to participate and the experience and expertise they contribute. (Hightower)

Park. She said these data served as an impetus for action to address health disparities.

In response to these stark data, as Hightower described, Rush embraced its role as an anchor institution.[1] Accordingly, the health system deployed its resources to intentionally and strategically invest in the West Side. This involved consideration of hiring practices, career paths, construction, supply chain, partnerships, procurement, investment in community economic development, and engagement of employees to volunteer in the surrounding community. In addition to using its own resources, by forming a collaborative, Rush could engage and persuade other health care institutions in the Illinois Medical District to make similar investments.

In partnership with the other anchor institutions, Rush developed the West Side Anchor Committee. In total, all partners involved had a combined 44,000 employees and supply chains worth more than $5 billion,

---

[1] Rush University Medical Center is a member of the Healthcare Anchor Network, supported through the Democracy Collaborative. See https://healthcareanchor.network/about-the-healthcare-anchor-network (accessed November 11, 2020).

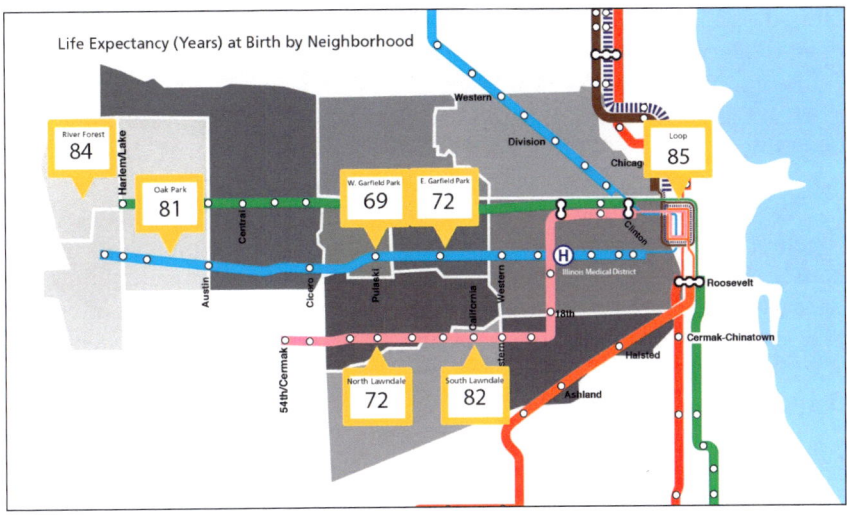

**FIGURE 4-1** Map portraying the average life expectancy (at birth) in Chicago neighborhoods by subway stop.
SOURCE: Hightower presentation, September 19, 2019.

which would make them the largest employer in the state of Illinois. The committee identified five key areas in which each of the anchor institutions would work:

1. Hire locally and develop talent.
2. Use local labor for capital projects.
3. Buy and source locally.
4. Invest locally.
5. Volunteer and support community building.

To elevate the anchor mission work within the health system and move it forward, Rush established executive leadership commitment and a new internal structure. Hightower concluded by pointing out that Rush's commitment served as a catalyst for other organizations operating on the West Side of Chicago, including community-based organizations, social services agencies, philanthropy, and government, which led to the establishment of West Side United.

## MANY VOICES: ONE WEST SIDE

Ayesha Jaco, West Side United, spoke about the West Side United coalition and the communities that it serves. As she explained, West Side

United spans 10 Chicago West Side communities that have historically been disenfranchised and experienced disinvestment because of historical racism and other factors. Many of the communities were devastated during the 1968 riots following the Reverend Martin Luther King, Jr.'s assassination and have not been rebuilt. Jaco asserted that these factors are key drivers of the current conditions in the communities.

West Side United has six collaborating organizations that came together to address community health and economic wellness in nearby communities on the West Side. The six participating organizations are Rush, which serves as the lead organization; Lurie Children's Hospital of Chicago; UI Health; Cook County Health; Sinai Health System; and AMITA Health. The collaborative has a shared vision of improving neighborhood health by examining inequities in health care, education, economic vitality, and the physical environment using cross-sector, place-based strategies.

Rush led the collaborative by bringing together partners to address the audacious goal of decreasing the gap in life expectancy by 50 percent between the Loop downtown and the 10 West Side communities depicted in Figure 4-1 by the year 2030. Jaco noted that it was important for Rush to ensure that the community was involved in the initiative. The health system did not want to create another prescriptive model that dictated to the community what it needed.

As Jaco described, Rush held listening sessions with community members from March through July 2017. Rush learned that community members wanted safe neighborhoods, access to care, equitable education, and jobs. Sixteen community members, half of whom were residents and half represented nonprofit and government entities, joined a planning committee to consider how to develop strategies. West Side United was officially launched in February 2018, when stakeholders from across the city convened to discuss plans for 10 initiatives. A leadership council, composed of executives and visionaries from the hospitals, was formed to guide the work and ensure support across the health systems. A small team of strategy, operations, and programmatic staff execute the agreed-upon strategies.

One key point made in the listening sessions drives the work of West Side United: "Nothing for us without us," meaning that nothing for the community should be developed without its involvement. A community advisory council, composed of 18 people who live or work in the community or represent nonprofit organizations based there, replaced the planning committee, which was dissolved 6 months after the establishment of the initiative. Jaco noted that in December 2018, six community advisory council members joined the six hospital chief executive officers on the leadership council.

West Side United has specific goals related to local hiring, which led the participating organizations to share hiring data for the first time. Participating organizations committed to hiring 3,500 people from the West Side by 2021, an increase from the 1,000 people currently employed. The coalition also launched employee career pathways to support advancement of nonclinical workers at the participating institutions. For example, one program supports an 18-month medical assistant pathway, with reimbursement for tuition and transportation provided.

Another example Jaco described is the Small Business Grant Pool, which was piloted in 2018 with $85,000 in total grants provided to support capital improvement and hiring of additional staff at seven small businesses. In 2019, a generous donation from JPMorgan Chase increased grant funding to $500,000 total for up to 30 grants, with the goal of helping to rebuild some of the communities that had not recovered since 1968.

Jaco used Figure 4-2 to describe West Side United's model. In the top left, storm clouds of systemic racism, disinvestment, and short-term focus create the current conditions. In the middle, community members build the bridge to overcome the challenges. At the bottom, institutions and partners build the pillars of the bridge.

In closing, Jaco used Figure 4-3 to describe West Side United's work from the perspective of residents and community organizations on one

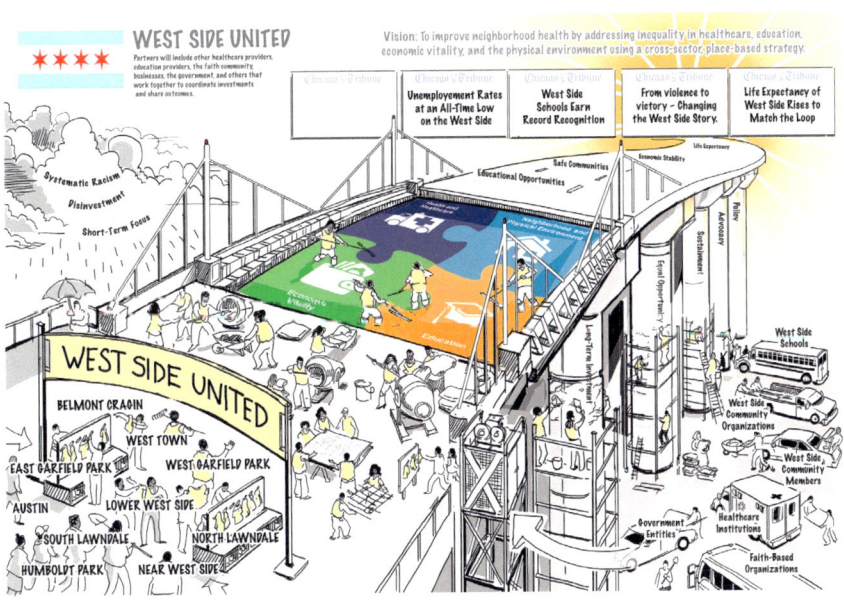

**FIGURE 4-2** A portrayal of West Side United's theory of change.
SOURCE: Jaco presentation, September 19, 2019.

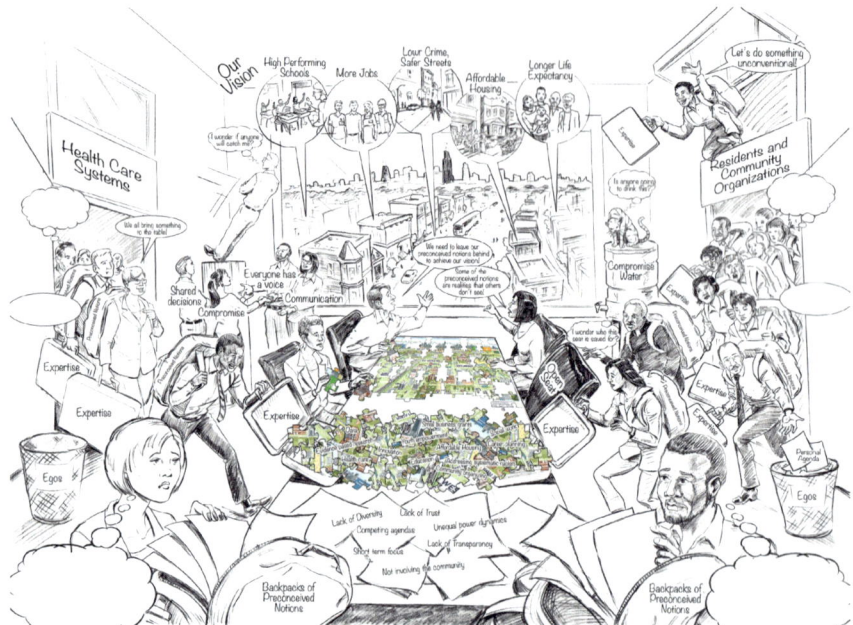

**FIGURE 4-3** A portrayal of West Side United's work with residents and community organizations and health care systems.
SOURCE: Jaco presentation, September 19, 2019.

side and health care systems on the other and how they work toward their shared vision of the community. On the resident and community organization side, people come to the table with their expertise, set their egos aside, and help to reformat the map. On the health care system side, health care systems come to the table as equal partners and work to build a shared vision for decreasing the gap in life expectancy.

## AUDIENCE DISCUSSION

Kraft opened the session's discussion period by saying "Change happens at the speed of trust." She asked Hightower and Jaco to describe successful practices for building trust between health systems and communities. Hightower responded that it is important for health systems to follow through on their commitments to communities, including showing up at events and providing grant funding. She emphasized the importance of shared decision making between health systems and communities, rather than health systems simply receiving feedback from community members. Jaco added that it is important for community members to have specific ways to participate that validate them as experts in their own experience, such as serving as ambassadors for their communities. She noted it is also helpful for other community members to see members of their community involved in the project leadership.

A participant asked Jaco about recommendations for getting health system executives into the community to understand the community's experience firsthand. Jaco answered in the affirmative, saying that the 18-member community advisory council includes representatives from all 10 West Side communities, each of whom have invited C-suite executives to be present in their communities. For example, a community tour could allow health system executives to better understand, appreciate, and support local communities by tasting their food, seeing the murals, interacting with residents, and learning about key organizations. As another example, health system leadership participated in an information session for the small business grants, which provided an opportunity for 170 small business owners in the West Side communities to interact with the health system leadership. Hightower also reiterated the importance of showing up to events when invited.

Building on the prior question, Jennifer Little of Klamath County Public Health in Oregon asked Jaco and Hightower how they train community members to feel prepared to speak with health system executives. Jaco responded that they engage community members based on their level of expertise. For example, those involved in education or small businesses participate in those subcommittees. They are also working with United Way to plan a training or fellowship for community members focused on development and diversity. She noted the importance of emphasizing that community members are experts and bring value to the discussion.

Wilkins added that it is equally important to provide orientation and set expectations for health system executives when working with community members. She suggested ensuring executives not only understand why community members want to speak with them but that they also understand the lived experience of the people in the community.

Marc Gourevitch of New York University Langone Health asked Hightower about the catalyst for institutional level change at Rush in 2015 that led it to decide to invest in improving health equity on the West Side and what the effect has been on the health system's bottom line. Hightower responded that the map in Figure 4-1 showing the differences in life expectancy between Chicago neighborhoods was a catalyst. In addition, David Ansell, Rush's former chief medical officer and current head of community health equity, had worked in safety net institutions on Chicago's West Side and had been focused on these disparities. With respect to the financial results, Hightower noted that Rush executives are excited about social impact investing because Rush will get a return on the approximately $4.5 million that has been invested to date, including reductions in emergency room visits by people on the West Side.

Ray Baxter of the Blue Shield of California Foundation asked about hospital labor unions' engagement in and support for the health equity work. Hightower responded that Rush has worked with the labor unions on employment pathways and other issues that affect union members.

Wilkins also commented on Rush's talent acquisition strategy, highlighting the importance of changing the culture by creating job descriptions that remove nonessential qualifications, such as a certain degree or a clean criminal record. Hightower added that pairing Rush's health equity work with its diversity and inclusion training could help to change the culture internally and build support for these changes in hiring practices. Jaco added that West Side United has helped to bring together hiring managers across the six participating institutions to consider ways to change policies.

Sanne Magnan of the HealthPartners Institute asked Hightower and Jaco about the most significant challenges they have faced in their work to date and what they see as future challenges. Jaco responded that a future challenge is community members' concern that they will not be able to afford to live in their neighborhood once improvements are made. She noted that the success to date has partly been attributable to the health institutions' intentionality and honesty about the role they have played in historically perpetuating—and more recently addressing—the disparities. She also emphasized the importance of having a well-known and well-respected champion such as Ansell, leveraging the power of the community, and bringing in resources from different sectors. Hightower added that she thinks the greatest future challenge is sustainably changing the culture to incorporate health equity in the long term. She is also concerned about how to lay the groundwork for continued funding for the work. Implementing the strategy in conjunction with institutional partners who were previously competitors and maintaining ongoing community relationships and support are also challenges.

# 5

# Midstream: Accountable Health Communities and Partnerships with Human Services Organizations

Session moderator Rahul Rajkumar of Blue Cross and Blue Shield of North Carolina introduced the panel by explaining that it would address how accountable health communities could serve as a model for partnerships between the clinical care delivery system and community service and human services organizations. Highlights from the two presentations and subsequent discussion are provided in Box 5-1.

Rajkumar began by giving some background on accountable health communities. He was previously on the staff of the Centers for Medicare & Medicaid Services' Center for Medicare & Medicaid Innovation (CMMI) when it launched the accountable health communities model, which he explained provides funding to "bridge organizations" for screening, referral, navigation, and encouragement of alignment (CMS, 2019). However, no CMMI funding may be used for community or social services. A forthcoming evaluation will determine whether the model will save the federal government health care costs.

## THE DENVER REGIONAL ACCOUNTABLE HEALTH COMMUNITY

A. J. Diamontopoulos of the Denver Regional Council of Governments (DRCOG) Area Agency on Aging began his presentation by explaining the concept of the accountable health community. As he described it, an accountable health community identifies people in a clinical setting who are high users of medical care (two or more emergency department visits in 1 year) and have unmet health-related social needs; it then refers them

> **BOX 5-1**
> **Key Points Made by Individual Speakers and Participants**
>
> - Health care funding for social services could allow such services to be increased, improved, and more targeted. (Diamontopoulos)
> - Improved integration between health care and community-based services provides the opportunity to address personal health needs holistically. (Scala-Foley)
> - Health care organizations prefer that contracting be centrally focused, a need that community-based integrated care networks can fill. (Scala-Foley)
> - Models such as accountable health communities may be useful in identifying gaps in availability of, and payment for, services that can help to address a person's holistic health needs. (Scala-Foley)
> - There is concern that social services could become overmedicalized with increased contracting between community-based organizations and health care organizations; community-based organizations need to balance the tension between being mission driven, data informed, and revenue generating so that they can continue to exist, innovate, better serve, and expand the populations they serve. (Scala-Foley)
> - Community-based organizations often serve as "eyes and ears," aware of the key issues in the community and how best to address them; it is important that these organizations emphasize their expertise and value when communicating with health care entities. (Diamontopoulos, Scala-Foley)
> - The fact that payment is available only for referrals—and not social services themselves—within the accountable health communities model poses a challenge. Social services need to be financially supported, and other issues and obstacles preventing those referred from accessing these services need to be addressed as well. (Scala-Foley)
> - Community-based organizations best serve people by meeting them where they are to be able to get them the services they need when they need them. (Sanchez-Warren)
> - The accountable health communities and other referral models may be useful in identifying which social services should be paid for by health care organizations and which may best be addressed through investment by nonmedical funders or broader policy change. (Auerbach)

to community-based organizations to get services to address these needs. He noted that ironically, this involves offering financial resources to the health care sector, which is often well resourced, to refer their patients to the social service sector, which is often underresourced.

As Diamontopoulos outlined, the DRCOG works on five health-related social needs:

1. Housing stability, such as homelessness or risk of homelessness, and housing quality, such as whether the home is clean and free of pests and mold;

2. Food security;
3. Utility needs;
4. Interpersonal safety, such as domestic violence, elder abuse, and child abuse; and
5. Transportation, which helps to connect people to services.

The primary goal is to integrate and align the screening and referral of Medicare and Medicaid beneficiaries from clinical to community services. The secondary goal is to reduce total health care costs and improve outcomes by addressing unmet health-related social needs by 2022.

Diamontopoulos described some of the challenges involved with screening people in a clinical setting and referring them to a community organization. As he explained, electronic health records have predetermined clinical settings and workflows that may not communicate with the systems at community organizations. Some community organizations also have their own privacy requirements. Others may not have the data systems in place that allow them to accept or send a secure electronic referral.

As Diamontopoulos explained, when the accountable health community model was launched in Denver in May 2017, clinical and community services providers had not previously worked with each other in a formal, structured manner. The first year was focused on development of a strategic plan, and the program got under way at the beginning of the second year. As part of the program, DRCOG is required to provide navigation services to a minimum of about 3,000 Medicare and/or Medicaid beneficiaries in six counties in the Denver area. DRCOG receives screening results from clinical partners, claims data from Medicaid, and community-level data from a small network of contracted partners. Once the data are received in full, it intends to conduct an analysis to understand the effect of the accountable health community model in the Denver region.

## PARTNERSHIPS WITH AREA AGENCIES ON AGING AND OTHER COMMUNITY-BASED ORGANIZATIONS

Marisa Scala-Foley of the National Association of Area Agencies on Aging (n4a) opened by explaining that her organization works to build the capacity of community-based aging and disability organizations to partner and contract with health care entities so that older adults and persons with disabilities can live in their communities for as long as possible. The work of the Aging and Disability Business Institute (the Business Institute) at n4a, which Scala-Foley oversees, is funded by The John A. Hartford Foundation, The SCAN Foundation, and the Administration for Community Living at the U.S. Department of Health and

Human Services, and is conducted in collaboration with other national and local organizations.

From Scala-Foley's perspective, the goal of the work of the Business Institute is to ensure that community-based organizations such as the Area Agencies on Aging that her organization represents are paid for the services they provide through contracts with health care organizations. n4a has fielded two request-for-information surveys to community-based organizations to learn more about the extent to which paid contracts exist.

As Scala-Foley explained, the survey found that the percentage of community-based organizations responding to the survey who had paid contracts to provide services or programs on behalf of or with a health care entity increased from 38 percent in 2017 to more than 41 percent in 2018. As Figure 5-1 shows, an increase in paid contracting was seen among centers for independent living, which serve people of all ages with physical disabilities; Area Agencies on Aging, which are "public or private nonprofit agenc[ies] designated by their state[s] to address the needs and concerns of all older persons at the regional and local levels" (ACL, n.d.); and other community-based organizations. The survey found the most common health care partners are Medicaid organizations, although

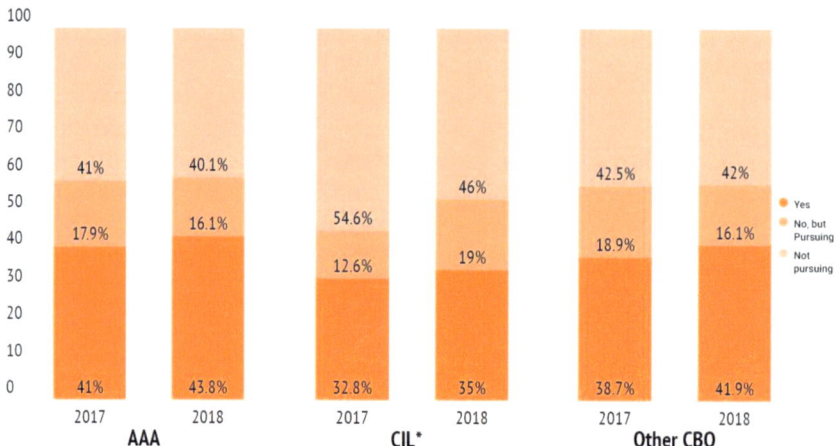

**FIGURE 5-1** Chart depicting the extent of paid contracts with health care organizations by type of disability and aging services organization in 2017 and 2018.
NOTES: AAA = Area Agencies on Aging; CBO = community-based organization; CIL = center for independent living. The data used in this graph were collected through a survey conducted by Scripps Gerontology Center at Miami University on behalf of the Aging and Disability Business Institute, led by the National Association of Area Agencies on Aging (n4a). For more information, visit http://bit.ly/cbo_contracts.
SOURCE: Scala-Foley presentation, September 19, 2019.

she expects that with changes to Medicare Advantage, contracts with Medicare Advantage plans will increase. As shown in Figure 5-2, top services provided include care coordination, care management, and service coordination, followed by care transitions, assessment of eligibility for long-term services, nutrition programs, and evidence-based health promotion programs.

Scala-Foley pointed out that health care organizations frequently comment that they do not want to have to contract with many small community-based organizations to serve a given geographic area and would prefer that their contracting be centrally focused. As a result, there has been an increase in community-based organizations doing business together as part of community-based integrated care networks. The survey found that in 2017, less than 20 percent of community-based organizations who were contracting with health care organizations did so through networks, but by 2018, that number had increased to more than

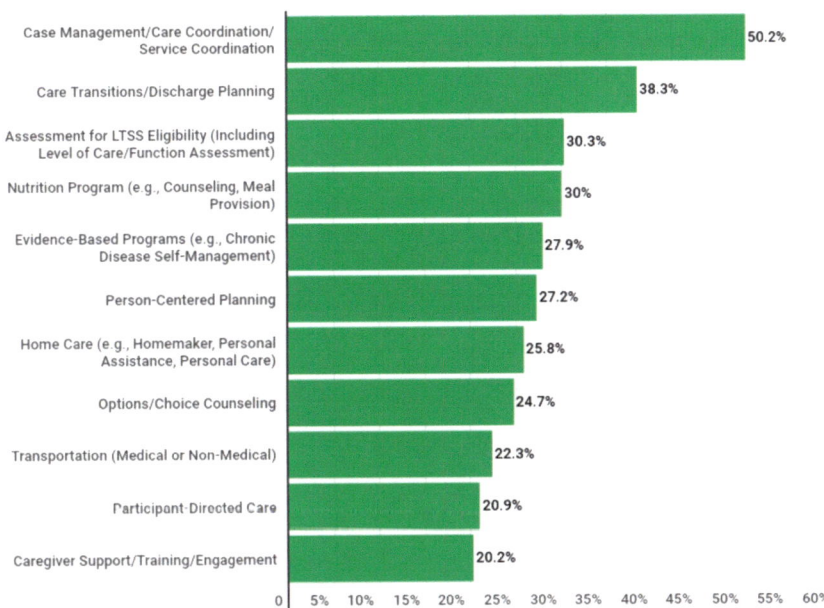

**FIGURE 5-2** Chart depicting the most common services provided by disability and aging services organizations through paid contracts with health care organizations. NOTES: The data used in this graph was collected through a survey conducted by Scripps Gerontology Center at Miami University on behalf of the Aging and Disability Business Institute, led by the National Association of Area Agencies on Aging (n4a). For more information, visit http://bit.ly.cbo_contracts. LTSS = long-term services and supports.
SOURCE: Scala-Foley presentation, September 19, 2019.

30 percent, a figure that Scala-Foley expects to continue to increase. Existing contracts tend to target high-risk, high needs groups.

A challenge with health care and community-based organization contracts that Scala-Foley highlighted is that health care and community-based organizations may not always use the same terminology or have the same attitudes toward issues. Diamontopoulos had also pointed out that the integration of social services referrals was a challenge.

## AUDIENCE DISCUSSION

Rajkumar opened the audience discussion by asking Diamontopoulos about the advantages and disadvantages of working with payers or entities engaged in the delivery of health care. Diamontopoulos responded that participating in the accountable health communities model was part of the strategy of the Area Agencies on Aging to obtain additional funding to help it meet the needs of the population it serves. He noted that a particular challenge is the "free rider problem" of health care entities not wanting to pay for services that the community-based organizations already provide "for free." However, Diamontopoulos pointed out that the work is not free and if health care entities provided funding, services could be increased, improved, and more targeted. A disadvantage of working with health care organizations is the time required to establish a contract. Diamontopoulos also noted the importance of community-based organizations emphasizing their expertise and value when communicating with health care entities.

Scala-Foley added that improved integration between health care and community-based services provides the opportunity to address a person's holistic health needs. As she stated, "Health happens in clinics and hospitals, but much more of it happens in homes and in communities." Scala-Foley further explained that since community-based organizations help to improve outcomes, and may help to generate cost savings, they should receive a share of those savings. While there has been payment reform in health care, community-based organizations addressing health-related social needs also need changes in their funding model, Scala-Foley asserted.

Rajkumar noted that the majority of the $3 trillion that the United States spends on health care is for care delivery funded through public payment systems (primarily Medicare and Medicaid) or health care premiums paid through employer-sponsored health insurance, taxes, exchanges, and fully insured products. He asked Diamontopoulos and Scala-Foley how they recommend communicating the value of community-based programs and services. Diamontopoulos responded that he thinks there will eventually be data showing that such services reduce health care costs. However, a challenge with this research is that there cannot be a control group that is denied social services. Diamontopoulos pointed out the research already shows that providing community-based services results in fewer emergency department visits.

Scala-Foley noted that her organization regularly communicates with community-based organizations about how to present their value proposition to different types of health care organizations. She agreed with Diamontopoulos that data resulting from existing contracts between health care and community-based organizations and other research studies are helpful. Scala-Foley and Diamontopoulos shared anecdotes about how community-based organizations are often the "eyes and ears" in the home, meaning they know what the key issues are in the community and how best to address them. Scala-Foley described the importance of matching the strengths of community-based organizations and the people they serve with the needs of a particular payer.

Rajkumar expressed concern that the evaluation of the accountable health communities model will not show an effect and asked Scala-Foley and Diamontopoulos for their recommendations regarding next steps in such a situation. Diamontopoulos responded that he agreed that such a result will be likely because referrals alone are not useful. As he explained, even if a need has been identified and a patient has been referred, no relationship has been built and the patient is unlikely to access the service. Diamontopoulos highlighted the point made by Laura Gottlieb in an earlier session that only a small number of people in need use community-based services. He speculated that this is not because people do not have the need, but rather because of the way the service is provided and the relationship, or lack of such, with the community-based provider. He emphasized the importance of targeting social services to people before they develop chronic medical conditions, and he said that it may take a long time (beyond 2022) to see results. Scala-Foley added that given that the accountable health communities model provides funds for navigation and referrals rather than the direct provision of social services, it may be useful in identifying gaps in availability of, and payment for, services that can help to address a person's holistic health needs.

Lourdes Rodriguez of the Dell Medical School at The University of Texas at Austin asked how to balance the need for deep knowledge of the communities being served with the need for uniformity of a single contracting mechanism. Diamontopoulos stated in response that the Area Agencies on Aging are the hub of a network of aging services providers. In contracting with a health care organization, they could either provide services or contract out through their usual channels. He further explained that last year his organization, DRCOG, brought approximately $14 million into the community through contracts to deliver services such as Meals on Wheels, transportation, and legal services. Scala-Foley added that there is also a concern that social services could be overmedicalized with increased contracting between community-based organizations and health care organizations. As she explained, social service organizations need to balance the tension between being mission driven, data informed, and revenue generating so they can continue to exist, innovate, better serve, and expand the populations they serve.

Bob Kaplan of Stanford University stated that about one-third of the money that health care payers give to provider groups, hospitals, and others are for services that do not make a difference. He hypothesized that this situation is unlikely to change because hospitals, provider groups, and payers—who have satisfactory medical loss ratios—are happy with the current arrangement. Diamontopoulos agreed that asking health care payers to invest in something outside of health care is challenging because they are not used to paying for such services. He suggested that incentives through quality measures, patient satisfaction scores, and regulatory change would be helpful in changing practices. He also pointed to the need for increased understanding that clinical care is one subset of health care, with community care and public health being additional components. As Diamontopoulos explained, spending on health care is unsustainable, with an expected $2 trillion in federal funds to be spent on Medicare and Medicaid just 7 years from now. In Colorado, spending on education and health care would make up the entire state budget. Diamontopoulos highlighted the need for increased education and awareness among federal and state lawmakers and insurance companies, who he noted are "paying for the most expensive kind of care."

Scala-Foley pointed out that changes in Medicare, including the addition of new benefits for chronically ill people in Medicare Advantage, may lead to additional changes in payment policies in Medicare fee-for-service and for private payers.

Jayla Sanchez-Warren of the DRCOG Area Agency on Aging, who works with Diamontopoulos, commented that the fact that the accountable health communities model does not allow for the payment of social services presents a challenge given the waiting lists for services. She noted that her organization had to obtain a grant from another organization to be able to provide services in conjunction with the new population that would need to be served with the accountable health communities grant. As Sanchez-Warren stated, "Referrals don't change health outcomes. Services change health outcomes." She further explained that a challenging aspect of the accountable health communities grant is getting people who are referred to come for services because they often face many other issues and have other priorities. For example, the people who are referred may not have the time to fill out a Supplemental Nutrition Assistance Program application or want to be asked the required questions. Those with chronic illnesses may be too tired to obtain and prepare food after a day of doctor's appointments. Sanchez-Warren highlighted the importance of meeting people where they are to be able to get them the services they need when they need them. For example, she noted that month-long waiting periods for services like Meals on Wheels are problematic.

John Auerbach, who was with the Centers for Disease Control and Prevention when the accountable health communities model was developed, stated that some of the expectation of screening patients for social needs was that the screening would identify needs and the health care institution would bring people together to discuss how to address them. He suggested that some of the discussion should involve consideration of which services should be paid for by health care and which may be best addressed by policy change or other nonmedical funders. For example, Auerbach explained that it was unrealistic to expect that the health care system would pay for affordable housing for every patient, but identification of the need for affordable housing could help to make the case that broader change is needed and bring policy makers to the table. Auerbach asked whether such conversations have taken place around the opportunities for funding streams from outside the health care sector.

Diamontopoulos responded that while he understands the theory behind the accountable health communities model, the variety of needs among the people the DRCOG Area Agency on Aging serves presents a challenge in its execution. For example, someone may need to prioritize addressing multiple needs, such as food, transportation, and utilities. As Diamontopoulos explained, someone who is food insecure may not have the energy to address utility challenges. He reiterated the need for increased education on the lack of investment in social services. However, Diamontopoulos suggested that health care organizations should make investments in social services such as food and housing, rather than become grocers or construction workers themselves.

# 6

# Upstream: Changing Environments, Changing Policy

Session moderator Lourdes Rodriguez of the Dell Medical School at The University of Texas at Austin introduced this session with a focus further "upstream" on opportunities for changing environments and policies as a way to improve population health. Highlights from the two presentations and subsequent discussion are provided in Box 6-1.

## POLICY AND ENVIRONMENTAL CHANGES TO IMPROVE HEALTH IN KLAMATH COUNTY, OREGON

Jennifer Little of Klamath County Public Health in Oregon began her presentation with a brief overview of Klamath County. As she explained, Klamath County is a rural county about the size of Connecticut with about 66,000 residents. It is located in south-central Oregon near the California border. While historically Klamath County was a logging community, the logging industry is no longer thriving, leading to high rates of poverty and a lack of living wage jobs. The county is newly focused on reinventing itself through recreation and renewable energy. The population is 78 percent white, 12 percent Hispanic, 4 percent Native American, and 4 percent mixed race, with nearly one in five people living in poverty.

Little stated that Klamath County is a health professional shortage area that struggles to retain health professionals. The lack of availability of clinical care makes it even more important to prevent chronic diseases and other illnesses. According to Little, Klamath County has done a lot with limited resources, relying heavily on partnerships and aligning resources in ways that maximize funding and staff capacity.

> **BOX 6-1**
> **Key Points Made by Individual Speakers and Participants**
>
> - Klamath County, in rural Oregon, has engaged in multiple partnerships and initiatives focused on improving healthy food access, physical activity, tobacco control, educational attainment, and access to health care. (Little)
> - Academic medical centers can use their respected voices to engage in upstream efforts to improve public health through educating decision makers, convening the medical community, and visibly stimulating policy change. (Cofer)
> - The University of Texas MD Anderson Cancer Center's engagement in a statewide Tobacco 21 policy in Texas provides a model for other academic medical centers to influence population health beyond their institutions. (Cofer, Hawk)
> - Compelling evidence, stories, and relationships are essential for advancing and implementing effective public health programs and policies. (Cofer, Hawk, Little, Rodriguez)
> - Academic health centers must consider the political environment and local context in selecting health policy proposals that they will promote or endorse. (Hawk)
> - Federal agencies could support or incentivize academic health centers to make an increased commitment to community action via regulations or funding. (Hawk)

Klamath County's focus on policy and environmental change began in 2012, when for the second year in a row the county was ranked at the bottom of the state in the County Health Rankings. Little noted that the county continues to be near the bottom. This ranking served as a call to action for the "core four" major health care players in the area: (1) the public health department; (2) Sky Lakes, the hospital system; (3) Klamath Open Door, the federally qualified health center; and (4) Cascade Health Alliance, the local Medicaid provider. To address the problem, the core four created a joint community health assessment and community health improvement plan. Each iteration of the plan since has been more focused and has involved more community partners. The Healthy Klamath Coalition was formed, which includes cross-sector representation from law enforcement, schools, local elected officials, the health care industry, and social services, Little explained.

As a result of their efforts, in 2018 Klamath County became a Robert Wood Johnson Foundation Culture of Health prize winner. Little pointed out that even though Klamath County is still near the bottom of the health rankings, the county is working toward better outcomes for all residents.

Little described several of Klamath County's health initiatives. The county has been particularly focused on improving food systems. As she explained, the Blue Zones Project health improvement framework recognizes that people spend the majority of their time within 5 miles of where they live. Such areas became the target for food system improvements. Klamath County wanted to take advantage of being an agricultural community and ensure access to products produced locally. The local food bank created an initiative called the Produce Connection, which had the initial goal of distributing 60,000 pounds of fresh produce throughout the community. The program was so successful that the following year they moved 600,000 pounds of produce. In 2018, the program distributed 1 million pounds of fresh produce through multiple distribution sites, including health care clinics, Special Supplemental Nutrition Program for Women, Infants, and Children (WIC) offices, job training program sites, and parks.

In addition, as Little explained, a food systems committee was established and the Klamath Farmers Online Marketplace was created, which operates as an online farmers' market in which producers such as ranchers, farmers, and beekeepers post their available products on a weekly basis and consumers reserve items for pickup. The county has a goal of making the marketplace more accessible to low-income residents. Supplemental Nutrition Assistance Program participants are able to use their benefits, although only a small number are taking advantage of the opportunity. The county is also considering how to increase fresh, healthy foods in its correctional facilities.

The Klamath Promise, Little outlined, is an initiative focused on increasing high school graduation rates. She noted that the county has poor graduation rates, largely because of chronic absenteeism. Some of the absenteeism, she pointed out, may be caused by health problems such as lack of dental care, illness, or parents who are unable to take time off from work to take their children to the doctor. The initiative is focused on reducing barriers to going to school, promoting high school graduation, or attainment of a GED. Little explained that the health department prioritized educational attainment because of its importance for health outcomes.

Klamath County has also engaged in changing tobacco control policy. As Little explained, the county has expanded access to tobacco cessation resources, is considering how to prevent youth from initiating tobacco use, and creating tobacco-free environments, including tobacco-free government properties, fairs, and parks. The county is also working on creating a tobacco-free downtown, although they have received some pushback from residents. Efforts to require tobacco retail licenses, which allows the government to regulate retailers and reduce sales to youth, have been successful. Little noted that because about one in three tobacco retailers had been found to be selling to youth, tobacco retailer education and enforcement is a priority.

The county aims to change the built environment to create more places for people instead of cars. For example, Little described, the county passed a complete streets policy and is working to improve connectivity of existing walking and bicycle routes. In addition, the mayor created a "10-Minute Walk Campaign" with the goal of ensuring that all county residents are within a 10-minute walk to a park. The local law enforcement has partnered with public health in improving park safety, and the hospital and Medicaid provider have invested tens of thousands of dollars to beautify and improve use of the parks.

Little concluded by describing a partnership between the public health department and the health system. The Oregon Health & Science University opened a rural campus in Klamath Falls, which includes a medical residency program and clinical students who complete rotations in the community. The program has increased access to health professionals including physician assistants, nurse practitioners, dietitians, and pharmacists, who also become involved in community health projects. Little expressed hope that the program will encourage some of the students to want to practice in rural areas like Klamath Falls.

## CHANGING THE ENVIRONMENT TO PROMOTE HEALTH OUTSIDE THE FOUR WALLS OF THE MD ANDERSON CANCER CENTER

Ernest Hawk and Jennifer Cofer of the University of Texas MD Anderson Cancer Center spoke about how their large cancer center is attempting to advance population health outside of the walls of its institution.

### MD Anderson's Cancer Control Strategy

Hawk began by explaining that MD Anderson is a traditional academic medical center involved in research, clinical care, and the education and training of future medical providers. However, for the past 40 years, the organization's mission has included a commitment to cancer prevention and control. To fulfill this part of its mission, MD Anderson dedicates about $25 million per year to prevention research, provides clinical preventive services in about 50,000 patient visits per year, and trains about 200 future health care professionals at a time. In addition, the organization is working to more simply define cancer control in language that can be understood by all 22,000 employees and to better execute its strategy.

As Hawk described, MD Anderson defines cancer control as evidence-based actions in three domains to effect meaningful, lasting, and measurable improvement at the population level outside of their clinical population. The three areas of action are policy, public and professional education outside of the institution, and services in the community beyond the institution walls.

One of MD Anderson's priorities outside the walls of their institution is reducing tobacco use, the leading cause of preventable death, disability, cancer incidence, and cancer mortality in the state of Texas. In addition, as Hawk highlighted, tobacco use is a modifiable risk factor that can be controlled with increased funding and resources. Therefore, MD Anderson has committed to using its resources and reputation to elevate the importance of reducing tobacco use both on its campus and in the surrounding community.

Hawk explained that to determine how MD Anderson would engage in tobacco control, 18 faculty members and staff with relevant expertise were convened, resulting in a lengthy document outlining evidence-based actions that had been taken by other tobacco control leaders at the population level. MD Anderson established three goals similar to those of the World Health Organization's (WHO's) Framework Convention on Tobacco Control (WHO, 2003). The goals are (1) reduce the prevalence of tobacco use at the population level, particularly among youth; (2) reduce the proportion of nonsmokers exposed to secondhand smoke; and (3) increase quit attempts by existing smokers.

To implement programs that address these three goals, MD Anderson relied on both internal research and the broader evidence base. The organization decided to operate at three levels: within its own institution, within its state and local region, and outside the state. Hawk concluded by describing the organization's broad approach to addressing tobacco control. This includes extension of a cessation program to providers outside the institution that has trained about 400 individuals. It also included work to establish tobacco-free policies in the 14 institutions across the University of Texas system. Previously, three of the campuses had no tobacco policy.

### MD Anderson's Engagement in Texas Tobacco 21

Cofer described MD Anderson's role in the Texas Tobacco 21 initiative as an example of how the cancer center has engaged in policy work. She noted that Tobacco 21 is a nationwide campaign to raise the tobacco sales age to 21, based on evidence stemming from a 2015 Institute of Medicine (IOM)[1] report that predicted such a policy would save lives, reduce lung

---

[1] As of March 2016, the Health and Medicine Division continues the consensus studies and convening activities previously carried out by the Institute of Medicine (IOM).

cancer, and reduce deaths (IOM, 2015). MD Anderson and other partners established and worked in a coalition for several years to educate lawmakers on the potential impact of a Tobacco 21 policy in Texas after similar legislation had been passed in other states.

After a failed 2017 attempt at a statewide policy, work began at the local level in San Antonio and surrounding areas. This involved forming a Texas Tobacco 21 coalition in partnership with other advocates. As a state institution and cancer center, MD Anderson was a respected voice, but restricted to serving in an educational capacity as a non-lobbying organization. Hawk provided testimony at committee meetings and other subject-matter experts met with legislators to educate them on the potential impact of the policy.

As Cofer explained, for MD Anderson to weigh in on a high-profile, impactful policy such as Tobacco 21, the organization had to have approval from its leadership, including the president, the government relations department, and the compliance and ethics division. Support for the policy also had to be cleared by the University of Texas System and Board of Regents, and it was adopted as one of MD Anderson's legislative priorities. The University of Texas System became a member of the coalition.

Cofer also outlined the many actions MD Anderson took to expand the Texas Tobacco 21 coalition from 13 to 100 partners in 2 years. As she explained, the coalition included diverse membership, with public health groups leading the advocacy efforts. Other partners included children's health groups, health systems, medical societies, statewide health and wellness associations and coalitions, the state association of business and local chambers of commerce, institutes of higher education, school districts, institutes for mental health and substance use, drug and alcohol coalitions, and health departments. Cofer noted that the nontraditional partners were particularly powerful messengers. As a state academic health center, MD Anderson's role was to engage health systems and coalition partners, participate in education at the community level, support press conferences and other visible activities and events with members of the medical community when asked, and garner the support of the medical community to promote the policy.

With respect to challenges, Cofer stated that working on a traditionally progressive public health policy in a conservative state led to difficulty in moving the policy through the legislative process. She noted that having champions among conservative leaders who were committed to reducing death and disease from cancer was particularly important. Reaching consensus on policy language among all coalition partners was also challenging. Ultimately, the Texas Tobacco 21 bill passed in May 2019 and was signed by the governor in June 2019, although Cofer acknowledged that some concessions were made in getting the bill passed.

In closing, Hawk noted that he was previously a program director at the National Cancer Institute, and federal agencies such as the National Institutes of Health and the Centers for Disease Control and Prevention can promote academic centers, such as cancer centers, making an increased commitment to community action. Hawk suggested that this could be done through regulations or funding.

## AUDIENCE DISCUSSION

Rodriguez opened the audience discussion by asking the panelists to describe a situation in which relationships between organizations or sectors helped to advance or hinder their public health work. Little responded that relationships are particularly important in a rural county with limited resources. For example, lack of clean, safe housing due to bedbug infestation and lack of housing overall are particular issues in Klamath County. To address the problems, the county established a Housing Task Force, including key stakeholders in areas such as public health, health care, economic development, and housing, to address how to encourage real estate investment and marketing. Little noted that the public health agency, the Medicaid program, and the housing authority are also jointly working on a proposal to create accountability regarding a response to the bedbug problem, obtain funding for the technology and service operators needed to remove the bedbugs, and provide tenant education regarding mitigation strategies. Little pointed out that the relationship is successful because the nontraditional partners trust each other's expertise.

Cofer added that the relationships of the coalition members with legislators and state leaders was the primary strength of the Tobacco 21 coalition. Different coalition members had relationships with different legislative champions. She also described how MD Anderson was able to enlist its Board of Visitors, a nonfiduciary, appointed advisory board of volunteers comprising business and community leaders who advance the institution's mission to end cancer, in the Tobacco 21 effort. For example, Board of Visitors members also educated state elected officials in a number of different settings outside the state capitol, such as social events back in their legislative districts. Hawk also described the importance of MD Anderson's relationship with other entities across the University of Texas System. As he explained, the 14 entities often did not know much about each other's priorities and viewed each other as competitors. Under the leadership of one of the University of Texas System leaders, representatives focused on population health from each of the 14 entities were convened on a quarterly basis, and each of the entities was tasked with developing a population health plan. Hawk noted that the result was a high-level blueprint for building relationships across the university.

Alyssa Crawford asked the presenters for their perspective on the types of research being done to influence policy makers or partners of the need for and type of action that should be taken and the best ways to communicate that evidence. With respect to Tobacco 21, Cofer noted that the evidence for the policy had already been marshalled in the 2015 IOM report (IOM, 2015), and The University of Texas at Austin had also conducted research on the impact of tobacco use locally. MD Anderson created a one-page infographic to explain the evidence and highlight the implications for Texas specifically, which it made available to other coalition members to also use in their education and advocacy efforts.

Hawk added that when MD Anderson decided to make a stronger commitment to prevention about 5 years ago, it began by compiling a database of its actions related to cancer control recommended by its researchers and other leading experts, such as WHO and the Community Preventive Services Task Force. To implement its cancer control strategy, MD Anderson hired staff with specific relevant expertise in implementing these types of policies and strategies. He noted that faculty were experts in implementation science and research but not necessarily implementation and dissemination itself. Hawk emphasized the importance of advocating for policies that are evidence based and having stories that support the policy and help to convince legislators of the need for action.

Little responded that while data is important to their work, getting access to local data can be challenging because there are no epidemiologists in Klamath County. She noted that the public health department relies heavily on the local university, which has a few professors willing to partner with and support them in gathering and analyzing data as needed. They also partner with the hospital system, but according to Little, it can be difficult to get the information needed from health care partners in a usable format. She also pointed out that legislators do not always understand that change in public health takes a long time, and an intervention may not be able to show results within a 1- to 3-year timeframe.

Marc Gourevitch commented that a health system such as MD Anderson engaging in public policy and working with partners at the state level is an ideal example of an upstream action to improve public health. He asked Hawk and Cofer if MD Anderson was considering engaging in similar efforts to affect other drivers of poor cancer outcomes, such as poor diet and physical inactivity. Hawk responded that it does plan to work on other issues, but it needs to consider the political environment in the state and choose policies that are appropriate for the context. He also noted that change takes time. For example, MD Anderson had been working to advance a comprehensive smoke-free law in Texas for 12 years, whereas they were successful in advancing a Tobacco 21 policy in just two legislative sessions. Cofer added that colleagues in her department are also engaged in place-based initiatives to address poor diet and physical inactivity in towns outside of Houston. She concluded with a call to action to challenge other cancer centers to engage in similar upstream efforts to improve public health.

# 7

# Small-Group Interactive Exercise: Up/Mid/Downstream Paradigms in Advancing Population Health and Health Equity

### INSTRUCTIONS

Lourdes Rodriguez of The University of Texas at Austin provided instructions for a small-group interactive exercise. Using the diagram shown in Figure 2-2 describing upstream, midstream, and downstream paradigms in advancing population health and health equity along with other axes for the conversation about addressing health-related social needs, participants were invited to work in small groups to exchange ideas and consider ways to move upstream in ways that are practical for their institutions. Participants also were asked to think about the tensions and promises and cross-cutting themes such as workforce, resources, policy, data, technology, and metrics highlighted in the panel sessions. To guide the conversation, participants were given the worksheet provided in Appendix C, which asks the following questions:

- What information does the diagram seem designed to convey?
- What are its possible uses?
- What changes are needed to make it more useful for specific audiences?
- How does this diagram help describe the role of my organization and work?
- How can I use this in my organization and in my work?
- How can I adapt this to describe my organization and my work?

After about 45 minutes, the workshop audience reconvened and several participants shared highlights from the discussion in which they had participated. These are summarized below. Statements, recommendations, and opinions expressed are those of individual participants and should not be construed as reflecting any group consensus.

## REPORT BACK

Reporting on one's group conversations, Mylynn Tufte of the North Dakota Department of Health shared that many participants found the diagram complete and that it appropriately conveyed cross-collaboration and cross-sector work. Some participants found it particularly useful for illustrating upstream efforts to establish policy, infrastructure, and systems for prevention and public health. They suggested that the diagram could be used to speak with decision makers, propose policies, and advocate for sustained funding. The group suggested that the diagram could be improved by adding columns for cross-sector collaboration and for resource needs. It could also be made more useful by considering the needs of patients, a key group not currently represented.

Other participants noted that the diagram conveys ways that organizations from all sectors could get involved in downstream, midstream, and upstream efforts to advance population health and health equity and move upstream. However, some pointed out that the diagram seemed largely focused on the health care sector. If this is the intended audience, they suggested more explicitly addressing issues in which the health care sector has a unique role to play, such as community benefit, community health improvement planning, anchor institutions, and employee wellness. With respect to intended uses, the group thought the diagram could be useful for helping organizations consider where they currently are with respect to addressing population health and health equity and the path forward. It could also be useful for mapping partners across sectors and for community health improvement planning. Regarding ways to improve the diagram, the group suggested it would be helpful for a future iteration to provide examples of sectors or potential partners in each area. In addition, they noted that some of the language is specific to the health care sector and changes to the terminology or framing could make it more useful for social service agencies or community-based organizations. The list of other relevant sectors could also be expanded to include those beyond health care, public health, education, and housing, such as criminal justice and the environment.

Several participants in another small group found the diagram potentially useful for educating and persuading leaders and decision makers and those outside of public health about strategies for advancing population health and health equity. Some suggested ways to make the diagram more useful for audiences outside of the health care sector, including noting the limited financial incentives for moving upstream. They also pointed out that community members and community-based partners such as faith-based entities and human services organizations such as the YMCA are missing from the diagram. Some participants suggested that the figure more clearly distinguishes between the distinct concepts of population health and health equity, the latter of which was perceived to be a component of the former. In addition, some participants underscored the importance of using language and terminology that resonates with the intended audience. To that end, they suggested using the terms *thriving* or *wellness* instead of *health*.

Presenting a last set of perspectives, Alyssa Crawford of Mathematica relayed a need to communicate a strong vision for population health that is not based solely on its history within health care. Some participants suggested that the diagram could be used as a tool for stakeholders and partners to consider the goals of their population health initiatives. The diagram, they added, could better convey the outcomes of population health initiatives and who will benefit from them. In addition, several participants noted that describing only upstream, midstream, and downstream interventions was limiting and did not adequately acknowledge the root causes of the population health challenges the interventions are intended to address, or the root causes of failure of population health efforts, such as lack of clear governance structures, communications, or infrastructure. Specifically, the diagram could better display the interconnectedness between upstream, midstream, and downstream interventions. Crawford also explained that contributors to the discussion suggested conveying incentives and accountability for each action, a suggestion that is especially important when multiple partners are involved. Some participants asserted that a picture, rather than a diagram, may better illustrate the logic model so it is more accessible to a less academic audience.

# 8

# Final Reflections

Joshua Sharfstein of the Johns Hopkins Bloomberg School of Public Health opened the final session of the workshop by sharing his reflections on the workshop.

Sharfstein commented that in recent years there has been an increased focus in health care on population health at all levels and the undertaking of activities that are more upstream—oriented toward policy change and systems change as opposed to individual clinical approaches. He noted that it is possible for the health care sector to be engaged in both downstream and upstream efforts and pointed to existing efforts by numerous organizations, including the Association of American Medical Colleges and the American Hospital Association. (See Box 8-1 for a series of questions that distill overarching individual speaker and participant observations and insights from the highlights boxes in each chapter.)

Sharfstein shared his three overarching points from the workshop. First, the workshop, he remarked, offered a map of the population health world, and it showcased the broadened understanding of population health. The map, in other words, is not uncharted territory, he said. Organizations and people have been working on these population health issues for a long time. He asserted that part of being successful is recognizing the work already taking place and collaborating with those already engaged. Second, Sharfstein suggested that it is acceptable for there to be multiple organizations working on an issue but there needs to be "order to the chaos," meaning there needs to be coordination and collaboration among stakeholders working toward similar goals. He sees providing coordination and structure as an important role primarily for public health. As

> **BOX 8-1**
> **Some Guiding Questions for Health Systems**
> **Distilled from Chapter Highlights**
>
> 1. Is addressing social factors a part of your health care practice and system?
> 2. Is your organization facilitating the necessary pathways for the community to be involved and invested in the design, implementation, and evaluation of the work?
> 3. How would you evaluate the level of trust between the community and your organization, and what can be done to improve it, if needed?
> 4. Does your organization have the internal coordination and communication that is a prerequisite to work with outside partners?
> 5. Is health equity a priority that is baked into the infrastructure, decision making, accountability, and other dimensions of your organization and the partnership in which it participates?
> 6. Is your organization engaged, as appropriate, in actions that can influence policy making upstream?
> 7. Is your organization considering the community effects of all of its business decisions, from procurement to investment?
> 8. Is your organization providing funding for and/or advocating for funding for social services and health-related social needs? (See the accountable health communities discussion in Chapter 5 about the model's promise and current limitations.)
> 9. What are some potential tools and strategies, including by federal agencies, to incentivize health system work in communities and to change the community conditions for health?

an example of building from downstream to upstream, Sharfstein traced the beginnings of Baltimore's work to improve early childhood outcomes to an effort and structure that was constructed to simply address safe sleep, and it has grown to encompass more than 100 organizations and a wide array of coordinated efforts. Third, he recommended focusing on activities that have meaningful goals and outcomes. A structure can be organized around an outcome. Sharfstein acknowledged being particularly struck by Little's comment that getting data can be difficult in some communities. He suggested that a role for health care could be to provide data that is helpful in informing cross-sector strategies.

Sanne Magnan of the HealthPartners Institute provided comments on the tensions and promise of the path upstream. She highlighted a tension that Laura Gottlieb of the Social Interventions Research and Evaluation Network at the University of California, San Francisco, raised of whether to invest in screening for social determinants of health versus addressing social determinants based on what is known about the patient's zip code.

Another tension that Magnan noted surfaced in the presentation from Darlene Oliver Hightower of the Rush University Medical Center: the sustainability of efforts to address social determinants of health. She also raised the issue of whether the health care sector, which already charges high prices for poor outcomes, should be tackling social determinants of health as a priority over high health care costs. She made the point that if health care costs were lowered, resources could be made available to invest in upstream approaches. Magnan clarified that her perspective is that health care organizations should both respond to rising health care costs and play a role in addressing the social determinants of health.

Robert Kaplan of Stanford University recalled three questions articulated decades ago about how to determine whether something works in medicine: Can it work? Does it work? Is it worth it? He noted that much of what the National Institutes of Health invests in is focused on answering the first question, using mouse studies and answering scientific questions under ideal circumstances. The second question of "Does it work?" is the basis of much of the work of the U.S. Food and Drug Administration. He noted that the third question is often left unanswered, with money being spent on health care interventions that may not be "worth it." As he explained, many clinical preventive services have small effects. For example, of 1,000 women screened with mammography, a high percentage of them will experience an adverse outcome, including the possibility of an unnecessary biopsy. Kaplan thinks addressing social determinants are clearly more "worth it" than clinical interventions, given the data presented on the differences in life expectancy and outcomes based on social factors such as geography. However, he remarked that the questions of "Can it work"? and "Does it work?" have not yet been adequately answered when considering addressing social determinants.

Marc Gourevitch of New York University Langone Health commented that much of the discussion at the workshop has been from the health care perspective, in keeping with the workshop design. He acknowledged Magnan's original framing that highlighted the tension over how population health may be overmedicalized by focusing on downstream close-to-the-patient solutions rather than upstream community and societal solutions effective at the population level. The day's presentations underscored the notion that the health care sector can do a lot to promote population health both on its own and in partnership. Gourevitch suggested that health care has the opportunity to play an even greater role without implying that there is not also a role for other sectors in addressing social and economic drivers of health. Gourevitch also recommended that public health agencies identify and assess progress toward measurable goals, such as increasing life expectancy by a certain amount within a certain number of years.

Mylynn Tufte of the North Dakota Department of Health commented about the tensions and promise of technology in improving population health. She noted that patients, consumers, health care providers, and payers all have expectations related to the use of electronic health records and smartphones.

A. J. Diamontopoulos of the Denver Regional Council of Governments Area Agency on Aging suggested that there is too much emphasis in health care on return on investment. Instead, he suggested that population health should be focused on doing what is right. Analogizing to the tech industry, Diamontopoulos pointed out that many of the major technology companies were not successful during their first 10 years, but many are profitable now. He suggested that if health care were to focus on doing what is right for the population it serves, then the return on investment will come.

Ernest Hawk of the University of Texas MD Anderson Cancer Center commented that he agreed with Diamontopoulos that health care workers get into the field to try to help people, and there is a need for increased emphasis on improving equity in addition to the more traditional metrics of safe, timely, and patient-centered care. He also highlighted the importance of data, suggesting that more inclusive and periodic assessment of health behaviors tightly correlated with health outcomes of interest would be particularly useful. He recommended both deeper and more frequent assessment in the communities with the greatest needs.

Philip Alberti of the Association of American Medical Colleges noted that there are uniquely American attributes that inhibit progress in population health and health equity. The values of individualism, competition, and racism get in the way of having effective coalitions that represent broad interests, he explained. He suggested that there is a need to better communicate with potential partners to understand what their own "selfish metrics" are for participating in the partnership, or in other words, how they or their organization will benefit. He suggested that effective partnerships should be able to achieve both individual and collective goals.

# Appendix A

# References

ACL (Administration for Community Living). n.d. *Area agencies on aging.* https://acl.gov/programs/aging-and-disability-networks/area-agencies-aging (accessed July 1, 2020).

Alderwick, H., and L. M. Gottlieb. 2019. Meanings and misunderstandings: A social determinants of health lexicon for health care systems. *Milbank Quarterly* 97(2):407–419. https://www.milbank.org/quarterly/articles/meanings-and-misunderstandings-a-social-determinants-of-health-lexicon-for-health-care-systems (accessed May 4, 2021).

Auerbach, J. 2016. The 3 buckets of prevention. *Journal of Public Health Management and Practice* 22(3):215–218.

Castrucci, B., and J. Auerbach. 2019. Meeting individual social needs falls short of addressing social determinants of health. *Health Affairs Blog.* https://www.healthaffairs.org/do/10.1377/hblog20190115.234942/full (accessed May 4, 2021).

CMS (Centers for Medicare & Medicaid Services). 2019. Accountable health communities model. https://innovation.cms.gov/initiatives/ahcm (accessed May 4, 2021).

Hessler, D., V. Bowyer, R. Gold, L. Shields-Zeeman, E. Cottrell, and L. Gottlieb. 2019. Bringing social context into diabetes care: Intervening on social risks versus providing contextualized care. *Current Diabetes Reports* 19(6):30. https://doi.org/10.1007/s11892-019-1149-y.

IOM (Institute of Medicine). 2015. *Public health implications of raising the minimum age of legal access to tobacco products.* Washington, DC: The National Academies Press. https://doi.org/10.17226/18997.

Kindig, D. A., and G. Isham. 2014. Population health improvement: A community health business model that engages partners in all sectors. *Frontiers of Health Services Management* 30(4):3–20. https://doi.org/10.1097/01974520-201404000-00002.

Lantz, P. M. 2019. The medicalization of population health: Who will stay upstream? *Milbank Quarterly* 97(1):36–39. doi: 10.1111/1468-0009.12363.

NASEM (National Academies of Sciences, Engineering, and Medicine). 2019a. *Integrating social care into the delivery of health care: Moving upstream to improve the nation's health.* Washington, DC: The National Academies Press. https://doi.org/10.17226/25467.

NASEM. 2019b. *Investing in interventions that address non-medical, health-related social needs: Proceedings of a workshop.* Washington, DC: The National Academies Press. https://doi.org/10.17226/25544.

WHO (World Health Organization). 2003. *WHO framework convention on tobacco control.* Geneva, Switzerland: WHO Document Production Services. https://fctc.who.int/publications/i/item/9241591013 (accessed May 4, 2021).

Woolf, S. 2019. Necessary but not sufficient: Why health care alone cannot improve population health and reduce health inequities. *Annals of Family Medicine* 17(3):196–199. https://www.annfammed.org/content/17/3/196.short (accessed May 4, 2021).

# Appendix B

# Workshop Agenda

Models for Population Health Improvement by
Health Care Systems and Partners:
Tensions and Promise on the Path Upstream: A Workshop

September 19, 2019
Location: Keck Center of the National Academies, Room 100
500 Fifth Street, NW
Washington, DC 20001

### WORKSHOP OBJECTIVES

1. Showcase main strategies (and the tensions and promise associated with them) for health care systems, blending leadership and partnership to address health related social needs, social determinants of health, and equity.
2. Explore and discuss the axes (and the tensions and promise associated with each) that frame the conversation: up, mid, and downstream; control and capability; social determinants of health versus health-related social needs; and advancing health equity across these axes.
3. Develop a framework that health systems, public health, community, and other sectors can use to situate and better understand the nature of their efforts—including both tensions and promise—to improve population health and promote health equity.

8:30 am     Welcome and Introductory Remarks

Sanne Magnan, Senior Fellow, HealthPartners Institute, Roundtable Co-Chair

8:45 am     Keynote Presentations: Overview of the Landscape; Tensions and Promise

Moderator: Marc Gourevitch, Chair, Department of Population Health, New York University Langone Health

Laura Gottlieb, Associate Professor of Family and Community Medicine, and Director, Social Interventions Research and Evaluation Network, University of California, San Francisco (via videoconferencing)
Benjamin Money, Deputy Secretary for Health Services, State of North Carolina

9:30 am     Discussion

10:00 am    Break

10:15 am    Panel I and Discussion: How Leadership and Organizational Structure Can Support Addressing Health-Related Social Needs and Advance Health Equity

Moderator: Philip Alberti, Senior Director, Health Equity Research and Policy, Association of American Medical Colleges

Consuelo H. Wilkins, Executive Director, Meharry-Vanderbilt Alliance; Associate Professor of Medicine, Vanderbilt University Medical Center and Meharry Medical College
Benjamin Carter, Executive Vice President and Chief Financial Officer, Trinity Health

10:55 am    Panel II and Discussion: Addressing Patients' Health-Related Social Needs ("Downstream")

Moderator: Sally Kraft, Vice President of Population Health, Dartmouth-Hitchcock

APPENDIX B 65

                Darlene Oliver Hightower, Vice President, Community Health Equity, Rush University Medical Center
                Ayesha Jaco, Senior Program Director, West Side United

11:35 am    Panel III and Discussion: Accountable Health Communities (and Partnerships with Human Services Organizations) as a Model ("Midstream")

                Moderator: Rahul Rajkumar, Chief Medical Officer, Blue Cross and Blue Shield of North Carolina

                A. J. Diamontopoulos, Accountable Health Communities Project Manager, Denver Regional Council of Governments Area Agency on Aging
                Marisa Scala-Foley, Director, Aging and Disability Business Institute, National Association of Area Agencies on Aging

12:15 pm    Lunch

1:15 pm     Panel IV and Discussion: Changing Environments, Changing Policy ("Upstream")

                Moderator: Lourdes Rodriguez, Director, Community-Driven Initiatives at Dell Medical School, The University of Texas at Austin

                Jennifer Little, Public Health Director, Klamath County, Oregon
                Jennifer Cofer, Director, EndTobacco Program, University of Texas MD Anderson Cancer Center, and
                Ernest Hawk, T. Boone Pickens Distinguished Chair for Early Prevention of Cancer, Professor of Clinical Cancer Prevention; Vice President and Head, Division of Cancer Prevention & Population Sciences, University of Texas MD Anderson Cancer Center

2:00 pm     Practical Small-Group Exercise and Report Back

                Moderator: Lourdes Rodriguez, Director, Community-Driven Initiatives at Dell Medical School, The University of Texas at Austin

3:30 pm    Final Reflections

           Joshua Sharfstein, Vice Dean, Johns Hopkins University
              Bloomberg School of Public Health, Roundtable
              Co-Chair

4:00 pm    Adjourn

# Appendix C

# Biographical Sketches of Presenters and Moderators[1]

**Philip Alberti, Ph.D.,\*†** is the senior director for health equity research and policy at the Association of American Medical Colleges (AAMC). Dr. Alberti supports the efforts of academic medical centers to build an evidence base for effective programs, protocols, and partnerships aimed at ameliorating inequalities in health and health care through research. Dr. Alberti is responsible for working with AAMC's constituents to elevate the status of community-partnered and health equity–related research efforts, identifying emerging funding sources and policy implications for such projects, and disseminating findings to achieve the broadest possible impact. Prior to joining AAMC in 2012, Dr. Alberti led research, evaluation, and planning efforts for a Bureau within the New York City Department of Health and Mental Hygiene that works to promote health equity between disadvantaged and advantaged neighborhoods. Dr. Alberti holds a Ph.D. in sociomedical sciences from the Columbia University Mailman School of Public Health and was a National Institute of Mental Health fellow in the Psychiatric Epidemiology Training program.

**Benjamin Carter, M.B.A.,** is the executive vice president, the chief financial officer, and the treasurer at Trinity Health. He has extensive knowledge of the organization, having led all aspects of the finance, treasury, risk management, revenue excellence, and payer strategies areas across the system. Additionally, he maintains operational responsibilities for

---

[1] * denotes planning committee member; † denotes roundtable member.

several ministries and has ongoing responsibility for integrating new ministries into the system.

Prior to joining Trinity Health, Mr. Carter served as the executive vice president and the chief operating officer of the Detroit Medical Center (DMC), where he was responsible for the operations of the regional system's eight hospitals and related outpatient facilities. During his tenure there, he was instrumental in DMC's financial turnaround, which resulted in 6 consecutive years of profitability. He led key growth, cost reduction, and profit initiatives in multiple service lines.

Prior to leading DMC operations, Mr. Carter spent nearly 17 years in executive-level positions at Oakwood Healthcare in Dearborn, Michigan. He started his career at Plante Moran in Southfield, Michigan, where he worked for 8 years.

Throughout his career, Mr. Carter has served on many internal and external boards including Care Tech Solutions, Inc., DMC Care Express, Invest Michigan Advisory Board, Boys Hope Girls Hope of Detroit, and was appointed the co-chair of Governor Rick Snyder's task force on Responsible Retirement Reform for Local Government. He is a member of the American Institute of Certified Public Accountants, the Michigan Association of Certified Public Accountants, and the Healthcare Financial Management Association. Mr. Carter is an alumnus of the University of Michigan in Ann Arbor, where he graduated magna cum laude with master's and bachelor's degrees in business administration.

**Jennifer Cofer, M.P.H.,** is the director of the EndTobacco Program and Cancer Prevention Policy at the University of Texas MD Anderson Cancer Center. Employing more than 18 years of experience in public health and tobacco control, she collaborates with internal and external partners to promote tobacco control initiatives and evidence-based best practices in policy, prevention, and cessation. She is a member of the American Public Health Association and the current chair-elect of the Cancer Alliance of Texas. Ms. Cofer holds a bachelor's in health education and an M.P.H., both from the University of Southern Mississippi. She has been a certified health education specialist for 20 years.

**A. J. Diamantopoulos** is the accountable health communities manager for the Denver Regional Council of Governments Area Agency on Aging. He leads the team working with clinical and community providers to demonstrate the critical link between better health outcomes and increased access to community-based services. Mr. Diamantopoulos earned a master's degree in health and health care policy from the University of Denver.

APPENDIX C

**Laura Gottlieb, M.D., M.P.H.,** is an associate professor of family and community medicine at the University of California, San Francisco (UCSF). A former National Health Services Scholar and safety-net family physician with fellowship training in social determinants of health, Dr. Gottlieb now serves as the principal investigator on multiple quantitative and qualitative projects examining the integration of social and medical care services. These projects range from large randomized trials on specific interventions undertaken in clinical settings to projects that explore the scope of this rapidly evolving field, including by characterizing the payment, technology, and workforce foundation for care integration. She is the founding director of the Social Interventions Research and Evaluation Network, a national research acceleration and translation institute supported by Kaiser Permanente and the Robert Wood Johnson Foundation (RWJF) that brings together researchers across the United States to synthesize, disseminate, and catalyze research at the intersection of social and medical care. Dr. Gottlieb is also the associate director of the RWJF National Program Office Evidence for Action grants program based at UCSF. She completed her M.D. at the Harvard Medical School and both her M.P.H. and residency training at the University of Washington. Dr. Gottlieb is affiliated with the UCSF Center for Health and Community.

**Marc Gourevitch, M.D., M.P.H.,†** is the Muriel G. and George W. Singer Professor and the founding chair of the Department of Population Health at New York University (NYU) Langone Medical Center. The focus of Dr. Gourevitch's work is on developing approaches that leverage both health care delivery and policy- and community-level interventions to advance the health of populations. Dr. Gourevitch leads initiatives in urban health metrics, is the co-director of the Community Engagement and Population Health Research Core of the Clinical and Translational Science Institute that bridges NYU Langone and New York City (NYC) Health+Hospitals, and leads NYU Langone's participation in the NYC Clinical Data Research Network funded by the Patient-Centered Outcomes Research Institute. His research centers on improving health outcomes among drug users and other underserved populations, integrating pharmacologic treatments for opioid and alcohol dependence into primary care, and developing strategies for bridging academic research with applied challenges faced by health care delivery systems and public sector initiatives. Dr. Gourevitch previously served as the founding director of NYU Langone's Division of General Internal Medicine and led NYU Langone's Centers for Disease Control and Prevention–funded Fellowship in Medicine and Public Health Research. A graduate of Harvard College and the Harvard Medical School, he trained in primary care/internal medicine at NYU and

Bellevue Hospital and received his M.P.H. from the Columbia University Mailman School of Public Health.

**Ernest Hawk, M.D., M.P.H.,** is the vice president and the division head for cancer prevention and population sciences at the University of Texas MD Anderson Cancer Center and holds the T. Boone Pickens Distinguished Chair for Early Prevention of Cancer. Additional responsibilities include leadership of the Duncan Family Institute for Cancer Prevention and Risk Assessment and co-leadership of MD Anderson's Cancer Prevention and Control Platform, which advances community health promotion and cancer control through evidence-based public policy, public and professional education, and community-based service implementation and dissemination.

A native of Detroit, Michigan, Dr. Hawk earned his bachelor's degree and M.D. at Wayne State University and his M.P.H. at Johns Hopkins University. He completed an internal medicine internship and residency at Emory University, a medical oncology clinical fellowship at the University of California, San Francisco, and a cancer prevention fellowship at the National Cancer Institute (NCI).

Prior to his appointment at MD Anderson in December 2007, Dr. Hawk held several positions at NCI in Bethesda, Maryland. He most recently served as the director of the Office of Centers, Training and Resources, responsible for NCI's cancer centers program, a major translational science program (i.e., the SPORE program), NCI's extramural training enterprise, and its extramural disparities portfolio. His prior NCI posts included the chief and medical officer in the Gastrointestinal and Other Cancers Research Group, the medical officer in the Chemoprevention Branch, and the chair of the Translational Research Working Group.

Dr. Hawk has been involved in a wide range of preclinical and clinical chemoprevention research, including developmental studies of nonsteroidal anti-inflammatory drugs, COX-2 inhibitors, and preventive agent combinations in high-risk cohorts. He earned numerous awards for his work, including the NCI Research Award for Distinguished Achievement in Cancer Prevention, the Distinguished Alumnus Award, and the American Society of Clinical Oncology/American Cancer Society Award. Most recently, his interests have broadened to include improvement of minority and underserved populations' participation in clinical research, and the integration of risk assessment, behavioral science, and preventive strategies developed through sequential clinical trials for application in clinical or public health settings. He has published more than 175 scientific articles and book chapters, edited 3 books, serves as the senior deputy editor for *Cancer Prevention Research*, and is on the editorial board of *Cancer Medicine*.

**Jessie Hecocta** is an enrolled member of the Klamath Tribes and is currently the relationship manager for the Blue Zones Project. Ms. Hecocta's education and passion for well-being has led her to become a team member of Blue Zones Project-Healthy Klamath. Ms. Hecocta has been driving the adoption of comprehensive well-being practices within a wide range of organizations for the Blue Zones Project since its launch in 2015. Ms. Hecocta's favorite principle from the Blue Zones Project is Right Outlook, which encompasses both downshifting and purpose; "taking the time to find your sense of purpose or best self takes quiet, reflection, and internal searching."

**Darlene Oliver Hightower, J.D.,** is responsible for the implementation and evaluation of community programs aimed to improve the health of individuals in the Rush University Medical Center's (Rush's) community areas. She oversees the Office of Community Engagement, which includes three school-based health clinics; Rush University community outreach programs, community benefit reporting, and Rush's cradle-to-career health care pipeline programs. Ms. Hightower is also a member of the senior leadership team for West Side United, a cross-sector, collective impact collaborative aimed at improving health and economic vitality on the West Side of Chicago. Prior to joining Rush, Ms. Hightower was the national vice president of programs for Public Allies, Inc. She is a Chicago Community Trust Leadership Fellow, a University of Chicago Civic Leadership Academy Fellow, and an Administrative Law Judge for the Chicago Department of Human Relations. Ms. Hightower attended Bradley University (graduating with high honors) and received her law degree from Georgetown University Law Center in Washington, DC.

**Ayesha Jaco** is a philanthropist, an educator, a choreographer, and the co-founder of M.U.R.A.L. (formerly the Lupe Fiasco Foundation). She has partnered with many Chicago-based organizations to provide comprehensive social services, substance abuse prevention, food equity, and study abroad and artistic programming for more than 18,500 inner-city youth and their families. In 2008, Ms. Jaco founded the youth dance company Move Me Soul and has provided more than 1,000 Chicago teens and young adults with professional dance training and life skill development.

Currently, Ms. Jaco is a faculty member at the Northeastern Illinois University Jacob Carruthers Center for Inner-City Studies. She was featured in *Hype Magazine South Africa* for her artistic prowess and youth work and she was recently awarded the Power 25 Chicago Award by Walker's Legacy for her commitment to excellent leadership, community achievements, and philanthropic contributions. Ms. Jaco holds a B.S. in dance and mass communication from Illinois State University and a master of arts management (arts in youth and community development) from Columbia College Chicago.

**Sally Kraft, M.D., M.P.H.,**\* is the vice president of population health at Dartmouth-Hitchcock, where she leads a multidisciplinary team dedicated to improving the health of populations and communities across the region served by Dartmouth-Hitchcock faculty and affiliates. She has worked with the High Value Healthcare Collaborative on disseminating evidence-based practices in health systems across the United States. Dr. Kraft served as the medical director of quality, safety, and innovation at the University of Wisconsin Health system from 2007 to 2014, where she led system-wide initiatives to redesign ambulatory care. She received her M.D. and M.P.H. from the University of Michigan, completed a residency in internal medicine at the Santa Clara Valley Medical Center, and fellowships in pulmonary and critical care medicine at Stanford University. She has practiced pulmonary and critical care medicine in Stanford, California, and Madison, Wisconsin.

**Jennifer Little, M.P.H.,** was born and raised in Fort Collins, Colorado. She earned a bachelor's degree in human development and family studies with a focus on healthy aging from Colorado State University. She then went on to earn her M.P.H. from Oregon State University. Ms. Little started her public health career as a tobacco prevention and education coordinator for Klamath County Public Health. She then worked for a nonprofit hospital system, Sky Lakes Medical Center, and helped develop a population health management program that utilized community health workers. Ms. Little then returned to Klamath County Public Health as the director. Ms. Little has a passion for public service and serves as the chair of the Community Advisory Council, the chair of the Blue Zones Project Built Environment Committee, and sits on the board of the Klamath Basin Senior Citizens' Center.

**Sanne Magnan, M.D., Ph.D.,**\*† is the co-chair of the Roundtable on Population Health Improvement of the National Academies of Sciences, Engineering, and Medicine. She is the former president (2006–2007) and the chief executive officer (2011–2016) of the Institute for Clinical Systems Improvement. In 2007, she was appointed the commissioner of the Minnesota Department of Health by Minnesota Governor Tim Pawlenty. She served from 2007 to 2010 and had significant responsibility for the implementation of Minnesota's 2008 health reform legislation, including the Statewide Health Improvement Program, standardized quality reporting, development of provider peer grouping, certification process for health care homes, and baskets of care.

Dr. Magnan was a staff physician at the Tuberculosis Clinic at St. Paul–Ramsey County Department of Public Health (2002–2015). She was a member of the Population-based Payment Model Workgroup of the Healthcare Payment Learning and Action Network (2015–2016) and a member of the Centers for Medicare & Medicaid Services' Multi-sector Collaboration Measure Development Technical Expert Panel (2016). She is on Epic's Population Health Steering Board and on Healthy People 2030 Engagement Subcommittee.

She served on the board of MN Community Measurement and the board of NorthPoint Health & Wellness Center, a federally qualified health center and part of Hennepin Health. Her previous experience also includes the vice president and the medical director of Consumer Health at Blue Cross and Blue Shield of Minnesota. Currently, she is a senior fellow with HealthPartners Institute and an adjunct assistant professor of medicine at the University of Minnesota. Dr. Magnan holds an M.D. and a Ph.D. in medicinal chemistry from the University of Minnesota and is a board-certified internist.

**Benjamin Money, M.P.H.,** joined the U.S. Department of Health and Human Services in 2019 as the deputy secretary for health services. Mr. Money previously served as the president and the chief executive officer of the North Carolina Community Health Center Association (NCCHCA), serving the 41 community health centers in the state. He led NCCHCA during a 10-year period of unprecedented growth in organizations, clinical sites, and patients served. In this role, Mr. Money was a member of the boards of the North Carolina (NC) Institute of Medicine, the NC Health Care Quality Alliance, the NC Health Information Exchange Advisory Board, the NC Safety-net Advisory Council, the Care Share Health Alliance, and the public health practice advisory committees for both the East Carolina Brody School of Medicine and the Gillings School of Global Public Health at the University of North Carolina (UNC) at Chapel Hill.

Mr. Money's 36-year career in health care began in community mental health and includes 11 years in local public health and 18 years with community health centers. He holds a master's degree in public health nutrition from UNC at Chapel Hill and he brings deep knowledge of health and North Carolina coupled with rich and varied leadership experience, passion, and vision.

**Rahul Rajkumar, M.D., J.D.,\*†** is the senior vice president and the chief medical officer at Blue Cross and Blue Shield of North Carolina (Blue Cross NC). Dr. Rajkumar came to Blue Cross NC after serving as the chief medical officer and the senior vice president for CareFirst BlueCross BlueShield. At CareFirst he developed and led programs addressing costs and health care improvement. These include initiatives related to model physician practices known as patient-centered medical homes, behavioral health, telemedicine, and substance abuse treatment.

Before joining CareFirst, Dr. Rajkumar served for 4 years as the deputy director of the Center for Medicare & Medicaid Innovation. He led federal efforts to promote value-based payments for physicians and hospitals, resulting in signing tens of thousands of agreements with providers worth billions of dollars. He also oversaw programs promoting primary care, the initial federal pilots for accountable care organizations, bundled payments for health care procedures, and patient safety initiatives.

Dr. Rajkumar has a bachelor's degree in history, a law degree, and a medical degree, all from Yale University. During his work at CareFirst and the federal government, he has worked as an attending physician at the Veterans Affairs Hospital in Washington, DC.

**Lourdes Rodriguez, Dr.P.H.,**[*][†] serves as the director of Community-Driven Initiatives at the Dell Medical School at The University of Texas at Austin. She works on community-engaged research and practice projects that build on ideas elicited from community colleagues. Previously, she served as a program officer at the New York State Health Foundation. From 2004–2012, she was a faculty member of the Columbia University Mailman School of Public Health. Dr. Rodriguez received a B.S. in industrial biotechnology from the University of Puerto Rico at Mayagüez, an M.P.H. from the University of Connecticut, and a Dr.P.H. from Columbia University.

**Marisa Scala-Foley, M.S.,** is the director of the Aging and Disability Business Institute at the National Association of Area Agencies on Aging, which provides community-based organizations with the tools and resources to successfully adapt to a changing health care environment, enhance their organizational capacity, and capitalize on emerging opportunities to diversify funding.

Recently, she served as the director of the Office of Integrated Care Innovations in the Center for Integrated Programs at the Administration for Community Living, where she managed the agency's efforts to build the capacity of state- and community-based organizations for delivery system reform. Before that, she helped found and lead the Center for Benefits Access at the National Council on Aging.

Ms. Scala-Foley has worked her entire career in the field of aging on issues related to health care and long-term services and supports. She holds a master's degree in gerontological studies from Miami University (Ohio) and a bachelor's degree in sociology/gerontology from the College of the Holy Cross in Worcester, Massachusetts.

**Joshua Sharfstein, M.D.,†** is the vice dean for public health practice and community engagement and a professor of the practice in health policy and management at the Johns Hopkins Bloomberg School of Public Health. He is also the director of the Bloomberg American Health Initiative. Previously, Dr. Sharfstein served as the secretary of the Maryland Department of Health and Mental Hygiene, as the principal deputy commissioner of the U.S. Food and Drug Administration, and as the health commissioner of Baltimore City. In these positions, he pursued creative solutions to longstanding challenges, including drug overdose deaths, infant mortality, unsafe consumer products, and school failure. He is an elected member of the National Academy of Medicine and the National Academy of Public Administration.

**Consuelo H. Wilkins, M.D., MSCI,** is the executive director of the Meharry-Vanderbilt Alliance and an associate professor of medicine at both the Vanderbilt University Medical Center (VUMC) and the Meharry Medical College. As the director of the Engagement Core of the *All of Us* Research Program (a component of the Precision Medicine Initiative), Dr. Wilkins oversees initiatives that meaningfully engage research participants in the governance, oversight, implementation, and dissemination of the program. She has pioneered methods of stakeholder engagement that involve community members and patients in all stages of biomedical and health research.

Dr. Wilkins is currently a principal investigator of two National Institutes of Health–funded centers: (1) the Vanderbilt-Miami-Meharry Center of Excellence in Precision Medicine and Population Health, which focuses on decreasing disparities among African Americans and Latinos using precision medicine, and (2) the Vanderbilt Recruitment Innovation Center, a national center dedicated to enhancing recruitment and retention in clinical trials. She is widely recognized for her work in stakeholder and community engagement and has pioneered methods of stakeholder engagement that involve community members and patients in research across the translational spectrum. One approach is the Community Engagement Studio—a model of engagement that can be used to elicit project-specific input from patients and communities at any stage of clinical or translational research.

Prior to joining the faculty at VUMC in 2012, Dr. Wilkins was an associate professor in the Department of Medicine, the Division of Geriatrics, with secondary appointments in psychiatry and surgery (public health sciences) at the Washington University School of Medicine in St. Louis, Missouri. She served as the founding director of the Center for Community Health and Partnerships in the Institute for Public Health, the co-director of the Center for Community-Engaged Research in the Clinical and Translational Science Awards Program, and the director of "Our Community, Our Health," a collaborative program with St. Louis University to disseminate culturally relevant health information and facilitate community–academic partnerships to address health disparities.

Dr. Wilkins serves on numerous boards and committees such as the National Academies of Sciences, Engineering, and Medicine's Committee on the Return of Individual-Specific Research Results Generated in Research, the American Association of Medical Colleges Journal Oversight Committee for Academic Medicine Laboratories, the Safety Net Consortium of Middle Tennessee, and the AcademyHealth Translation and Dissemination Institute Advisory Committee. Dr. Wilkins is an invited speaker around the country and a mentor to many junior faculty and health professions students.

# Appendix D

# Small-Group Exercise: Up/Mid/Downstream Paradigms in Advancing Population Health and Health Equity

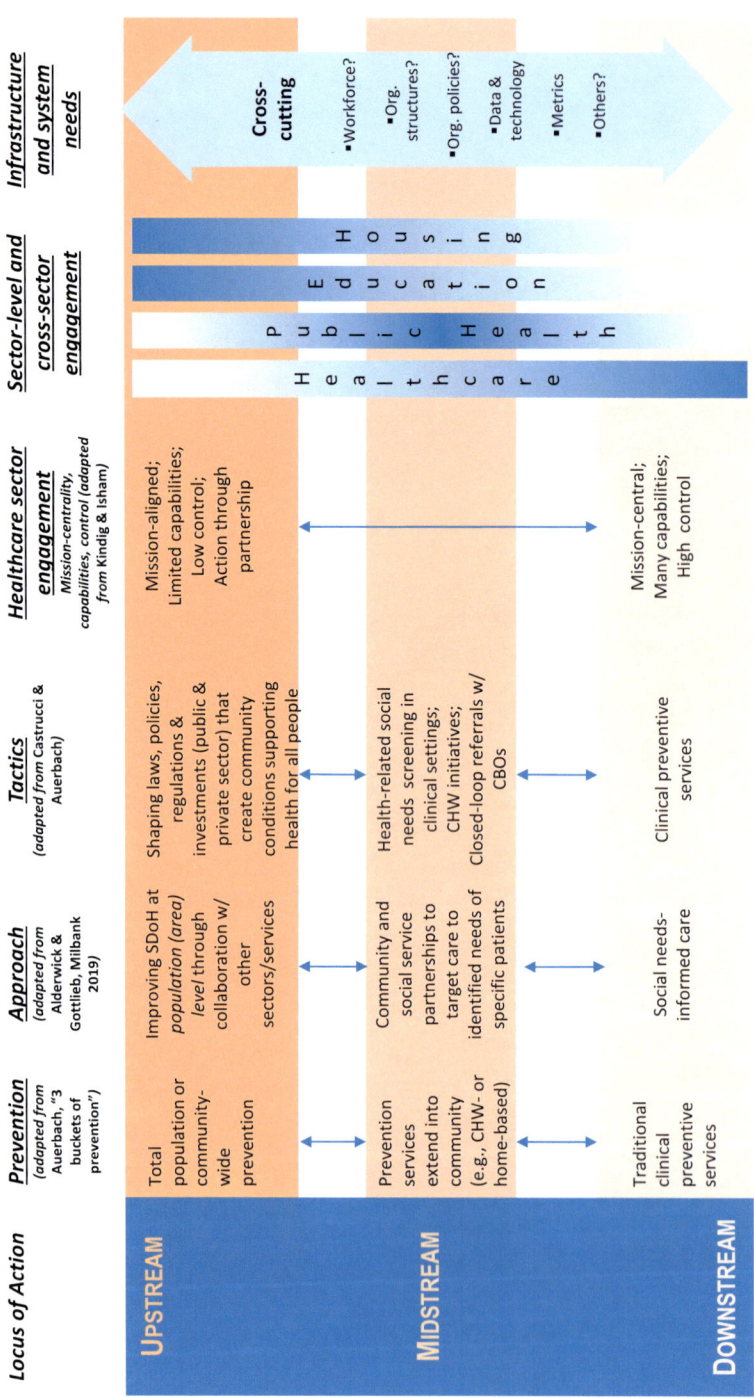

## WORKSHEET FOR THE PRACTICAL EXERCISE
### Toward Co-Creating Shared Language to Understand and Advance Population Health and Health Equity

(1) Identify a rapporteur and a note-taker; annotate the large format version of the diagram, to report group feedback and leave behind for NASEM staff; Keep the handout for your reference, and to continue the conversation after today.
(2) Reflect on the presentations and discussion of the day, and the tensions and promise of upstream approaches to advance population health. Considering the Cross Cutting Needs: Workforce, Organizational Structures & Policies, Data & Technology, Metrics and any other considerations, review the diagram and answer the following questions.
(3) For comments from the web, email abaciu@nas.edu.

| What information does the diagram seem designed to convey? | How does this diagram help describe the role of my organization & work? |
|---|---|
| What are its possible uses? | How can I use this in my organization, my work? |
| What changes are needed to make it more useful for specific audiences? | How can I adapt this to describe in my organization, my work? |

*References:*
Castrucci, B, and J Auerbach. 2019. Meeting Individual Social Needs: Falls Short of Addressing Social Determinants of Health. Health Affairs Blog.
Kindig, DA, and G Isham. 2014. Population Health Improvement: A Community Health Business Model That Engages Partners in All Sectors. Frontiers of Health Services Management.
Auerbach, J. 2016. The 3 Buckets of Prevention. Journal of Public Health Management and Practice.
Alderwick, H, and LM Gottlieb. 2019. Meanings and Misunderstandings: A Social Determinants of Health Lexicon for Health Care Systems. Milbank Quarterly.